Coronary Care

WILLIAM E. BODEN, M.D.

Director, Coronary Care Unit
The Miriam Hospital

Assistant Professor of Medicine
Brown University
Providence, Rhode Island

ROBERT J. CAPONE, M.D.

Director, Coronary Care Unit
Rhode Island Hospital

Associate Professor of Medicine
Brown University
Providence, Rhode Island

Foreword by

Herbert J. Levine, M.D.

Chief, Cardiology Division
New England Medical Center

Professor of Medicine
Tufts University School of Medicine
Boston, Massachusetts

W.B. SAUNDERS COMPANY

Philadelphia London Toronto
Mexico City Rio de Janeiro Sydney Tokyo

W. B. Saunders Company: West Washington Square
Philadelphia, PA 19105

1 St. Anne's Road
Eastbourne, East Sussex BN21 3UN, England

1 Goldthorne Avenue
Toronto, Ontario M8Z 5T9, Canada

Apartado 26370—Cedro 512
Mexico 4, D.F., Mexico

Rua Coronel Cabrita, 8
Sao Cristovao Caixa Postal 21176
Rio de Janeiro, Brazil

9 Waltham Street
Artarmon, N.S.W. 2064, Australia

Ichibancho, Central Bldg., 22-1 Ichibancho
Chiyoda-Ku, Tokyo 102, Japan

Library of Congress Cataloging in Publication Data

Boden, William E.

Coronary care.

Includes index.

1. Heart—Infarction—Treatment. 2. Coronary heart disease—Treatment. 3. Coronary care units. I. Capone, Robert J. II. Title.

RC685.I6B57 1984 616.1′23206 83–17161

ISBN 0–7216–1072–2

Coronary Care ISBN 0-7216-1072-2

Last digit is the print number: 9 8 7 6 5 4 3 2

To our wives, Barbara and Emilie,
with deep gratitude for their patience,
encouragement, and support.

FOREWORD

It is now 20 years since the coronary care unit (CCU) was introduced to the practice of medicine. During that time, the management of patients with acute coronary heart disease has changed from a passive and expectant approach to a dynamic scene in which the attitude of the physician is to "seek and destroy" the threat of adversity. Sophisticated systems for arrhythmia detection are now universal, and the capability of hemodynamic monitoring of pulmonary pressures and cardiac output is fast becoming routine in community hospitals everywhere. While this intensive approach to acute coronary care has proved expensive and is not without some risk of its own, the inpatient mortality of acute myocardial infarction has almost *halved* in two decades. Although part of this benefit is likely related to a multiplicity of factors, there is good reason to believe that modern acute coronary care has resulted in a substantial saving of lives.

The prompt use of antiarrhythmic agents and, when necessary, DC cardioversion and defibrillation has virtually eliminated death from primary ventricular tachyarrhythmias in the CCU. The introduction of balloon-tipped, flow-directed catheters into the right heart chambers has provided clinicians with quantitative bedside measurements of pressure and flow that guide our therapy of power failure and pulmonary congestion. The utility of this information is perhaps best illustrated in the care of patients with right ventricular infarction, in whom accurate serial measurements of right heart and pulmonary capillary pressures are crucial to achieving optimal therapy. Rupture of the interventricular septum can be quickly differentiated from papillary muscle rupture or dysfunction, and most importantly, the effects of pharmacologic interventions can be assessed with simplicity and speed, and in serial fashion.

In addition, the recent introduction of percutaneous intraaortic balloon insertion not only has increased the speed and availability of intraarterial counterpulsation to patients with acute coronary heart disease but also has created a new role for the cardiologist in the surgical treatment of this disease. Indeed, in many institutions, the CCU is now part of a network that involves the catheterization laboratory and the operating room.

These developments have placed an extraordinary burden upon the physicians and nurses in the CCU. The exploding technology of catheters, introducers, intraaortic balloons, pacemakers, and so on, and the burgeoning clinical pharmacology of an ever-increasing number of antiarrhythmic agents, inotropic drugs, adrenergic blockers, calcium channel blockers, and fibrinolytic agents inevitably has forced the CCU team to keep abreast of the recent, almost logarithmic growth of medical and technologic information.

In this setting, the book *Coronary Care* by Drs. Boden and Capone will find a ready audience for health care professionals in the CCU and will provide them with timely and extremely useful information. The text is concise yet comprehensive, up-to-date, and organized so as to permit quick access to the "nuts and bolts" of coronary care. While the handbook includes considerable background data, the major value of the volume is the practical discussion of diagnostic and therapeutic decision points, "how to" information regarding invasive procedures, methods of administration and doses of cardiac drugs, and identification of pitfalls and iatrogenic problems that may confound the efforts of the CCU team. This text deserves a place in every CCU and will prove an extremely useful reference for all who care for patients with acute coronary heart disease.

HERBERT J. LEVINE, M.D.

PREFACE

The purpose of this *Coronary Care* handbook is to review comprehensively the spectrum of acute ischemic heart disease as it relates to the patient who is admitted to the CCU with suspected myocardial infarction. This book was written in response to numerous requests from cardiology fellows, house staff, nurses, and paramedical professionals who sought a thorough, organized, yet readable account of the many diagnostic and therapeutic facets that comprise coronary care.

The handbook is structured in five major sections:

(1) A discussion of relevant clinical and pathophysiologic information pertaining to acute ischemic heart disease, *before* the CCU;

(2) An in-depth discussion of the CCU-hospital phase, which details such pertinent issues as emergency management of the acute infarct patient, CCU orders, diet, activity, the diagnosis and prognosis of myocardial infarction;

(3) Invasive monitoring for the CCU patient, a section devoted to hemodynamic monitoring, pacemakers, and intraaortic balloon counterpulsation;

(4) The treatment of myocardial infarction and angina pectoris and their complications; a comprehensive discussion of the pharmacologic management of acute infarction, unstable angina, cardiogenic shock, and other adverse sequelae of myocardial infarction; and

(5) A brief discussion of the recovery phase postmyocardial infarction beyond the CCU, including cardiac rehabilitation and "step down," or progressive care telemetry unit monitoring for arrhythmia surveillance.

We have included at the end of some chapters a few pertinent references. These are intended to provide review sources for a more in-depth treatment of the topic or to serve as an initial source of information on new topics not well covered in the standard texts.

WILLIAM E. BODEN, MD
ROBERT J. CAPONE, MD

ACKNOWLEDGMENTS

We are indebted to Richard S. Shulman, M.D., Physician-in-Chief at The Miriam Hospital, and Albert S. Most, M.D., Chief of Cardiology at The Rhode Island Hospital, for their scholarly guidance and support.

We are grateful to Patricia Hatch for her expert assistance in the preparation of the illustrations and for her help in designing the book cover. Among the many individuals who have given their devoted secretarial efforts to the preparation of this manuscript, we would like to acknowledge Diane Scott, Sally Lafreniere, Constance Arvanites, Christine Abatiello, and Janice Bordieri.

We would like to thank Albert Meier, Editor-in-Chief of W. B. Saunders Company, for his initial approval of and enthusiastic support for this project, and members of his staff, in particular Wynette Kommer, Bill Preston, Terri Siegel, and John Dyson. Mr. Dyson especially provided the behind-the-scenes guidance, encouragement, and professional services befitting his role as Medical Editor of the Blue Book Series.

We wholeheartedly express our gratitude to all these individuals.

William E. Boden, M.D.
Robert J. Capone, M.D.

CONTENTS

PART IV CCU TREATMENT OF MYOCARDIAL INFARCTION, ANGINA PECTORIS, AND THEIR COMPLICATIONS

INTRODUCTORY NOTE

The Saunders Blue Books Series is intended to provide, in a handy, convenient format, up-to-date information about therapy and patient care across a wide range of clinical fields. Blue Books are designed to help practicing physicians, nurses, emergency personnel, and other health care professionals and students to deliver quality patient care. Our series derives its title from the very first W. B. Saunders publication (Hare: *Essentials of Physiology,* Saunders, 1888). This book was part of a famous list of 24-question compends known as the "Blue Series." The purpose of that series was to sort out important scientific and clinical facts so that students could review and assess their knowledge. The name of the present series reflects its heritage from that pioneering venture. Today, when scientific information is growing exponentially, health professionals recognize an increasing obligation both to remain current and to select from this sea of facts those that add significantly to that foundation upon which sound clinical practice is based. The Blue Books address this need. They should not be regarded as textbooks or office references, but as portable clinical tools—as vital to quality patient care as a stethoscope or blood pressure cuff.

MICKEY S. EISENBERG, M.D., PHD.
Consulting Editor, Blue Books Series

I

BEFORE THE CCU

1
INTRODUCTION

Coronary artery disease may cause no symptoms at all, or it may evoke myocardial ischemia that is clinically manifested as angina pectoris, arrhythmias, myocardial infarction (MI), congestive heart failure (CHF), or sudden death. Ischemic heart disease, therefore, can present as a spectrum—from no symptoms to clinical expressions of intense pain or discomfort. The basis for myocardial ischemia and its relationship to coronary artery disease will be discussed in subsequent chapters.

The syndrome of angina pectoris that Heberden described in 1768 is still an effective and accurate model. The term *angina pectoris* probably stems from the Latin "angor animi," which means suffocation. Rather than using the word "dolor," which simply means pain, Heberden attempted to characterize the sense of strangulation or oppression that he observed often to accompany his first cases of chest (or rather "breast") pain:

"They who are afflicted with it, are seized, while they are walking (more especially if it be uphill and soon after eating) with a painful and most disagreeable sensation in the breast, which seems as if it would extinguish life, if it were to increase or continue, but the moment they stand still, all this uneasiness vanishes." Thus, Heberden, in his original report, described many of the features that are still associated with this symptom complex: episodes of pain that are paroxysmal in nature, are often related to effort (such as walking or eating a large meal), and are relieved promptly by rest.

Dr. Paul Wood's classic writings on angina pectoris provide a suitable, systematic framework for characterizing it: (1) *character,* (2) *site and distribution,* (3) *provocation,* and (4) *duration.*

The *character* of angina pectoris may be described as shortness of breath with a sense of constriction around the larynx or upper trachea. A characteristic feature is the often crescendo increase in intensity of the anginal pain, which is followed by a gradual fading away of the sensation. Certain descriptive features of chest discomfort militate against its being of myocardial ischemic origin. Angina is seldom described as "sharp or stabbing" or as "catching"; rarely is it affected by changes in posture or by deep breathing.

In describing the chest discomfort, the angina patient frequently indicates a *sizeable area of involvement* with the whole hand or clenched fist (positive Levine sign). The designation with a single finger to a specific point on the chest is unusual in classic angina pectoris. Radiation of the pain is not essential for the diagnosis, but radiation to the upper extremities, particularly the inner aspects of the left upper arm and forearm, is helpful in excluding certain other possible causes. Clearly, left arm radiation is not specific for angina pectoris, since this may be observed in cervical radiculitis or other musculoskeletal conditions. On the other hand, radiation of pain or discomfort to the jaw, teeth, or face is more specific for angina pectoris but is relatively infrequent.

The *precipitating factors* in angina pectoris are usually effort, emotion, cold weather, or eating a heavy meal. However, in some individuals, chest discomfort may occur at rest and, if it is typical in character, may indicate progression of coronary artery disease, such as the development of unstable angina (see Chapter 22).

Anginal pain is usually a few minutes in *duration,* with extremes occurring from 30 seconds to 30 minutes. Shorter or longer durations are unusual in angina pectoris. The prompt relief of discomfort following sublingual nitroglycerin is often helpful in the diagnosis, but several trials may be required before the pattern can be conclusively established, and this is not entirely specific for the diagnosis of ischemic heart disease, since other conditions (such as reflux esophagitis, hiatus hernia, gastritis) may likewise respond to nitroglycerin. The effect of nitroglycerin is generally apparent within 1 to 2 minutes. It is emphasized that severe attacks of angina pectoris may not respond even to several sublingual nitroglycerin tablets; this event may herald impending myocardial infarction.

Angina pectoris may be the first clinical manifestation of coronary artery disease. Approximately 40 per cent of new coronary events in men and 60 per cent of new coronary events in women are angina attacks that are unassociated with myocardial infarction. This group of patients generally has "stable angina pectoris." In contrast, angina pectoris also may appear shortly before or sometimes after a myocardial infarction. Such "periinfarct" angina, or "unstable" angina, is twice as common in men as in women. Approximately 50 per cent of men and 15 per cent of women with angina pectoris have had a myocardial infarction in the past.

Myocardial infarction (MI), or ischemic necrosis of the myocardium, is due to interruption or severe compromise of the myocardial blood supply. A severe manifestation of coronary artery disease, it not only causes many deaths but also almost invariably compromises left ventricular function and occasionally results in intractable congestive heart failure ("power failure") with a poor prognosis. Almost all instances of MI are atherosclerotic in origin, although nonatherosclerotic causes (coronary arterial spasm, connective tissue disorders, hemostasis disorders, or defects in platelet agglutination that occur in some patients who use oral contraceptives) have been described.

The characteristic clinical feature that dominates the presentation of myocardial infarction is severe, prolonged chest discomfort, which is often associated with restlessness, anxiety, and a fear of impending death. The pain generally has the same distribution and radiation as that of angina pectoris, but usually it is more intense and protracted, persisting often for 30 or more minutes.

The initial episode of pain associated with acute myocardial infarction typically subsides within a few hours and, except for some residual soreness, almost always abates within 24 hours. When chest pain persists beyond the first day or recurs within the first 4 or 5 days, a diagnosis of extending myocardial infarction, or unstable angina, is made unless pericarditis is present or pulmonary embolism has occurred.

In contrast to angina pectoris, MI as a rule is not precipitated by effort; rather, more than half the cases occur during sleep or rest and only 2 per cent during unusual effort. As stated, MI may develop either as a new event in an otherwise asymptomatic individual (in male patients, 50 per cent of new coronary events are MIs) or in patients without antecedent angina pectoris.

A substantial number (15 to 20 per cent) of patients develop so-called "silent" or asymptomatic myocardial infarction, as revealed by routine serial electrocardiograms. In addition, a significant number of MIs are dominated by symptoms of dyspnea, congestive heart failure, atypical pain location, shock, and cerebrovascular accidents (so-called "anginal equivalents"), with pain being minimal or absent.

Sudden coronary death accounts for 50 to 60 per cent of all deaths attributed to coronary artery disease. In patients with symptomatic coronary disease, 40 per cent of all deaths are sudden; among individuals dying suddenly with severe coronary artery disease but no other cause to explain the death, 60 per cent have no antecedent anginal symptoms. Approximately one quarter of victims who succumb suddenly had reported some warning symptoms (angina, dyspnea, fatigue, indigestion) on the day of death. Risk factors associated with sudden coronary death have not been clearly defined, but it does appear that cigarette smoking is strongly related. Hypertension and ECG evidence of left ventricular hypertrophy are also significant contributors; serum lipid and lipoprotein changes do not appear to be associated with sudden death (see Chapter 3).

The mechanism of sudden death is overwhelmingly arrhythmogenic. Ventricular fibrillation occurs in about three quarters of cases, while asystole ("cardiac standstill"), high-grade atrioventricular block, and ventricular tachycardia make up the remaining 25 per cent.

The prevention of sudden cardiac death is *the* major preventive health care challenge in this country today. Approximately *one million deaths* are due to coronary disease in the United States annually, of which 500,000 to 600,000 occur *prior to,* or shortly after, admission to the hospital. The early hospital phase of myocardial infarction (including the prevention of sudden death due to arrhythmias) will be discussed in detail in Chapter 3.

REFERENCES

Braunwald E (ed): Heart Disease: A Textbook of Cardiovascular Medicine. 1st ed. Philadelphia, W. B. Saunders Company, 1980, p 1387.

Heberden W: Some account of a disorder of the breast. Med Trans R Coll Physicians *2*:59, 1972.

James JN: Chance and sudden death. J Am Coll Cardiol *1*:164, 1983.

Wood P: Diseases of The Heart and Circulation. 3rd cd. Philadelphia, J. B. Lippincott, 1950, p 2.

2

PATHOPHYSIOLOGY OF MYOCARDIAL ISCHEMIA AND THE CORONARY CIRCULATION

Myocardial infarction (MI), or ischemic necrosis of the left ventricle, is the end result of the irreversible deprivation of nutrient blood flow and oxygen supply to cardiac muscle. The fundamental thesis of the supply-demand ratio is critically important to the understanding of myocardial hypoxia (decreased oxygen delivery) and ischemia (decreased blood flow or coronary malperfusion), which are the pathophysiologic basis for infarction (necrosis or death of viable cardiac muscle tissue).

Traditionally, coronary thrombosis had been considered the major cause of acute myocardial infarction. However, this belief has been challenged, and alternative hypotheses have been postulated:

- hemorrhage or rupture of an atherosclerotic plaque, producing coronary occlusion;
- coronary arterial spasm;
- excess myocardial oxygen requirements in relation to compromised perfusion through chronically (and critically) stenosed vessels, leading to periods of diminished coronary blood flow;
- platelet or fibrin plugging;
- elaboration of vasoactive substances such as thromboxane.

Whatever the exact mechanism(s), it appears certain that, in almost all cases, atherosclerotic narrowing of the coronary arteries is the principal progenitor of coronary occlusion, regardless of the ultimate event; coronary thrombosis is associated, either as a primary or secondary event. Atherosclerosis results from the chronic accumulation and inclusion of lipid in the vessel wall. This is believed to be due to the presentation of elevated levels of serum lipids to the subendothelial arterial spaces, either as a result of a break or a tear in the endothelial arterial spaces, or a result of increased levels of cholesterol in the blood itself (i.e., hypercholesterolemia), or both.

The introduction of lipids into the cells of the arterial wall appears to largely depend on the low-density lipoprotein (LDL) moiety. Elevated serum levels of total cholesterol, particularly the LDL fraction, appear to facilitate the process of atherosclerosis. The increased amount of blood cholesterol may be due to secondary (dietary) factors; or to primary factors, such as genetic familial

Table 2–1. SUPPLY

Supply may be reduced with
1. Fixed coronary narrowing
2. Dynamic obstruction (spasm) alone or superimposed on No. 1.
3. Heart rate: With increases, the duration of diastolic coronary flow to the left ventricle decreases
4. Coronary "steal"
5. Coronary perfusion gradient: The difference between aortic diastolic and left ventricular diastolic pressures. Decreased aortic pressure and/or raised LVEDP narrow the gradient for coronary perfusion.

predispositions; or to aberrations in intracellular LDL receptors. Hypertension enhances the entrance of lipids, although few researchers regard it as the sole or major initiating factor in the development of atherosclerosis. As such, it is felt to be additive as a risk factor with elevated blood lipids in the development of atherosclerosis (see Chapter 3).

Why certain arteries, such as those in the coronary or cerebral circulation, seem particularly prone to the development of atherosclerotic lesions is unclear at present. Moreover, why women are "protected" until menopause from developing a high incidence of coronary events is likewise unknown, although recent studies suggest that in addition to hormonal factors, higher serum levels of "protective" high-density lipoprotein (HDL) may be responsible for this phenomenon in premenopausal women, as well as other groups such as vegetarians, runners, and joggers.

Since myocardial ischemia is related to an imbalance between myocardial oxygen supply and demand, the management of patients with ischemic heart disease is predicated on the recognition and correction of this imbalance, either by increasing the capacity of the coronary arteries to supply blood to ischemic myocardium or by reducing the myocardial oxygen demand. The specific therapeutic regimens for treating myocardial ischemia are based on the *medical management* of coronary artery disease, which is aimed primarily toward reducing myocardial oxygen **demand,** and its *surgical management,* which is designed to improve myocardial blood flow and oxygen **supply** (i.e., increasing nutritive blood flow to areas supplied by obstructed coronary vessels) via direct myocardial revascularization, utilizing aortocoronary saphenous vein bypass grafts or by dilating the stenosed coronary artery (percutaneous transluminal coronary angioplasty, PTCA).

Coronary blood flow: The major determinant influencing myocardial oxygen supply (Table 2–1)

The major limitations of coronary blood flow are due to fixed atherosclerotic lesions, which narrow the coronary artery lumen. Coronary flow becomes critically limited when the obstruction exceeds 70% of the coronary arterial luminal diameter (50% when obstruction involves the left main coronary artery).

Dynamic obstruction, due to coronary spasm, may occur in any coronary anatomic location, may vary in intensity from time to time, and may increase the severity of a given stenosis from partial to complete.

Heart rate, in large measure, determines the duration of coronary blood flow, especially in the setting of ≥ 70% coronary luminal narrowing. The majority of nutritive coronary blood flow occurs during diastole; to the extent that heart rate is inordinately accelerated (tachycardia), the duration of diastole will be correspondingly shortened, and flow will be attenuated.

In the presence of a significant coronary obstruction, a reduction in the resistance to flow in an *adjacent* coronary artery vascular bed may divert blood flow away from an already ischemic area ("coronary steal"). Such an unfavorable shunting of blood flow may be caused by drugs that preferentially dilate coronary arterioles (resistance vessels), such as nitroprusside, hydralazine, and certain calcium-channel blockers, such as nifedipine.

Increases in LVEDP (and left ventricular volume) will increase ventricular wall tension and may compress the coronary arterioles in the subendocardium, producing a decrease in myocardial blood flow to this region. Similarly, reductions in the driving force of this blood flow (coronary perfusion pressure), a direct consequence of aortic diastolic pressure, may decrease myocardial blood flow. Thus, the difference between aortic diastolic pressure and LVEDP is known as the gradient for coronary perfusion; factors that decrease aortic pressure (hypotension) or increase LVEDP (myocardial failure)—alone or in combination—will narrow the gradient and reduce net myocardial blood flow.

Myocardial oxygen consumption: The major determinant of myocardial oxygen demand (Table 2–2)

Myocardial oxygen consumption has three major determinants and three minor determinants. The major determinants are systolic ventricular wall stress, heart rate, and myocardial contractility (the strength and vigor of myocardial contraction).

Ventricular wall stress is directly related to ventricular cavitary size (volume), intraventricular pressure, and wall thickness during systole.

Heart rate increases myocardial oxygen consumption largely by increasing the number of ventricular contractions per minute. In addition, heart rate governs not only the duration of that systolic wall stress or tension but is inversely related to the duration of diastole, which is the time in the cardiac cycle during which the

Table 2–2. DEMAND

Major Determinants:
- Heart rate: ↑ chronotropy accelerates $M\dot{V}O_2$ and intensifies ischemia
- Contractility: ↑ inotropy in the nonfailing heart may ↑ $M\dot{V}O_2$
- Myocardial wall tension
  - Afterload
  - Preload

Minor Determinants:
- Myocardial fiber shortening
- Activation energy
- Peripheral basal metabolic requirements increased by:
  - Fever
  - Hypovolemia, anemia
  - Thyroid, catecholamine excess

majority of coronary blood flow is delivered to the left ventricle. As the heart rate increases, the duration of diastole shortens, and the duration for nutrient coronary flow likewise shortens. Tachycardia increases myocardial oxygen consumption ($M\dot{V}O_2$) and can intensify ischemia.

The *contractile state* of the myocardium (contractility) is the third major factor that determines the amount of oxygen expended by the myocardium for any given level of work.

The three minor determinants of myocardial oxygen consumption are peripheral basal metabolic requirements, the activation of contraction, and myocardial fiber shortening (see Table 2–2).

Therefore, $M\dot{V}O_2$ increases when left ventricular systolic pressure, volume, or wall thickening increase; when the heart rate becomes elevated; when the contractile state of the myocardium is enhanced (either endogenously because of increased sympathetic catecholamine elaboration or exogenously because of drug administration, such as digitalis or synthetic cathecholamines); and when there are increased peripheral metabolic requirements, such as fever or thyroid excess. Any derangement of the above parameters can adversely affect the myocardial supply-demand ratio and produce (or worsen) myocardial ischemia. This delicate balance in supply and demand (changes which mediate the development of myocardial ischemia) is depicted graphically in Figure 2–1.

Finally, the time course of myocardial ischemia and infarction is the subject of considerable debate and continuing controversy (see Chapter 24). Myocardial infarction surely results when some myocardial cells receive insufficient nutrient blood flow and oxygen. However, other myocardial cells, both adjacent to and somewhat remote from the center of ischemic necrosis, are rendered severely ischemic by the same process that caused the MI. It is generally

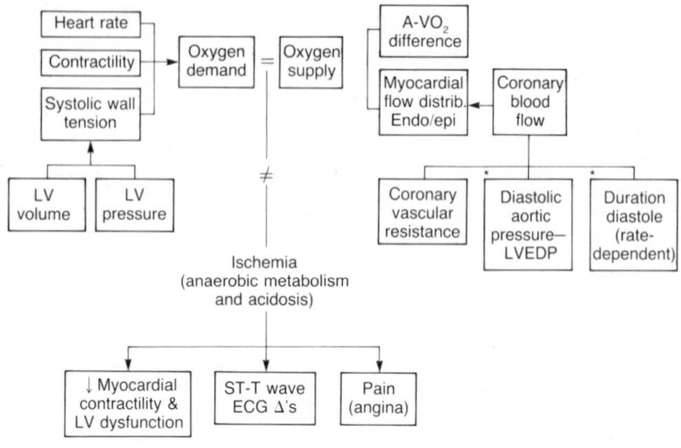

Figure 2–1. Flow chart summarizing the relationship between factors influencing myocardial oxygen supply and demand. Under normal conditions, diastolic aortic pressure and heart rate (duration of diastole) do not govern coronary blood flow, since blood supply is "autoregulated" at the arteriolar level (i.e., changes in coronary vascular resistance modulate coronary blood flow). In the presence of coronary arterial narrowing (≥ 70% luminal diameter reduction), the major determinants of flow (*) become the diastolic perfusion pressure (aortic diastolic pressure—diastolic ventricular filling pressure) and heart rate. Such imbalances in oxygen supply or demand result in myocardial ischemia, which is clinically manifested by angina, ECG changes, or abnormalities of left ventricular function. (From Sonnenblick EH, Frishman WH: The role of beta-adrenergic blockers in the treatment of angina pectoris. Cardiovasc Rev Rep *2*:442, 1981.)

held that damage to the latter cells is not irreversible or homogeneous; rather, there may be a heterogeneous population of less severely ischemic cells in a "border zone" around the central infarct that are jeopardized but not yet necrotic. This "border zone of jeopardized myocardium" has become the focus of modern coronary care basic and clinical research, which directs therapy to reduce infarct size and decrease the likelihood of developing myocardial pump failure (see Chapter 20). Most interventions that reduce the demand of myocardial cells for nutrients (especially oxygen) will be beneficial to this jeopardized ischemic myocardium. Specific therapeutic regimens that either enhance myocardial blood flow and oxygen supply or reduce myocardial oxygen consumption ($M\dot{V}O_2$) will be discussed in detail in Chapters 16–20.

REFERENCES

Cohn PF, Vokonas PS: Pathoanatomy and pathophysiology of coronary artery disease, *in* Diagnosis and Therapy of Coronary Artery Disease. Cohn PF (ed): Boston, Little, Brown, 1979, p 227.

Gould KL: Dynamic coronary stenosis. Am J Cardiol *45*:286, 1980.

Gregg DE, Patterson RE: Functional importance of the coronary collaterals. N Engl J Med *303*:1404, 1980.

Klocke FJ: Measurements of coronary blood flow and degree of stenosis: Current clinical implications and continuing uncertainties. J Am Coll Cardiol *1*:31, 1983.

Marcus ML: The Coronary Circulation in Health and Disease. New York, McGraw Hill, 1983.

3

PREHOSPITAL CORONARY CARE

THE ACUTE EVENT

Definition

Prehospital coronary care is that therapy given a patient with presumed acute myocardial infarction in the interval between the onset of symptoms and arrival at the Emergency Room. Prehospital mortality ranges between 40 and 60% and occurs chiefly within the first hour after the onset of symptoms. Early studies have suggested that a well-organized prehospital system, operating under medical direction and providing routine cardiac care as well as Advanced Cardiac Life Support, can markedly reduce this mortality (Crampton et al). Attempts to decrease patient and physician delay and thereby achieve the full benefit of this approach have been instituted in some communities. Citizen-initiated cardiopulmonary resuscitation (CPR) has also been found effective in reducing prehospital mortality (Cobb et al).

Diagnosis

Diagnosis should be largely based on history, since ECG abnormalities may not be present in the early phases of acute myocardial infarction, or the ECG may show only hyperacute changes (peaking of T waves in the involved area). Therapy, therefore, should not await the arrival of ECG, defibrillator, or telemetry equipment.

Treatment

Considered here is therapy by the physician or nurse in a prehospital setting. Recommendations for paramedic protocols are well provided elsewhere and are not within the scope of this chapter.

For All Patients:

(1) Reassurance of all conscious patients

(2) Treatment of pain. This may be the most efficacious measure in the patient with suspected acute myocardial infarction. **Nitroglycerin** has been increasingly used for the initial treatment of pain. It is particularly recommended for this purpose if pain has been present for less than 30 minutes, even if the patient has already taken nitroglycerin. It has the advantage of possessing fewer cardiac

vascular and respiratory depressant effects compared with morphine and may limit cardiac muscle damage.

Hypotension or tachycardia, both undesirable if excessive, may occur with nitroglycerin use. These adverse effects are seen primarily in the volume-depleted patient; nitroglycerin should be used in such patients only with caution or not at all. Should blood pressure fall rapidly or to 90 mm Hg or less or should heart rate rise above 100, the patient's feet should be raised or the patient should be placed in the Trendelenburg position.

Recommended dose: 0.4 mg sublingually. If systolic pressure remains above 100 mm Hg, the dose can be repeated in 5 minutes if moderate or severe pain persists.

Alternatively, **morphine sulfate,** 4 mg IV (subcutaneously if IV route not easily attained) may be given. Additional IV dose increments of 2 mg may be given every 5 minutes as needed, to a total of 8–10 mg. Morphine generally should not be given to those with chronic respiratory disease or others susceptible to respiratory depression.

(3) Oxygen administration by mask at 4–6 L/min. Patients with evidence of chronic lung disease should receive oxygen at lower concentrations (1–2 L/min) and then only with physician or nurse surveillance.

For Those with Symptoms Suggestive of MI Without Complicating Arrhythmias or Impaired Hemodynamics:

(1) *Ventricular arrhythmia prophylaxis*: Lidocaine, 75 mg IV. One or two additional 50 mg bolus doses given every 5–10 min may be advisable to reach prophylactic levels. Each bolus should be given slowly over 90 sec. There is conflicting evidence regarding the efficacy of lidocaine given by a standard IM technique; 300 mg IM had been recommended in the past but found ineffective by some investigators for preventing life-threatening ventricular arrhythmias.

(2) *Prevention of sinus bradycardia:* Initial studies showed a high incidence of autonomically mediated sinus bradycardia during the early stage of acute MI; the bradycardia was effectively treated with atropine. Later studies have failed to confirm the frequency of this arrhythmia. Moreover, treatment in the absence of hypotension or other signs of hypoperfusion may result in sinus tachycardia with aggravation of myocardial ischemia. Therefore, neither prophylactic therapy nor therapy of asymptomatic bradycardia is recommended. Should hypotension or signs of hypoperfusion be evident when the heart rate is below 50 beats/min, 0.5–1.0 mg of atropine IV should be given.

For Those with Symptoms Suggestive of MI and with Ventricular Arrhythmias (in Absence of Heart Failure or Shock):

Lidocaine, 75 mg IV initially, then 50 mg every 5 minutes until relief of the arrhythmia or until 225 mg is given. *Remember:*

Lidocaine will not alter supraventricular arrhythmias. In the absence of ECG recording by standard equipment or radiotelemetry, premature beats detected by pulse or stethoscope should be considered as ventricular in origin.

For Those with Symptoms Suggestive of MI and with Heart Failure:
(1) *Furosemide* (Lasix), 40 mg IV, or *nitroglycerin* (sublingual or cutaneous) may rapidly relieve congestive hemodynamics by lowering preload. In the congested patient without shock, there is little chance of these agents producing hypotension.

(2) *Arrhythmia prophylaxis*—as noted for ventricular arrhythmias; after the initial 75 mg dose, however, decrease subsequent doses by 50%. Maximum dose, 125 mg.

For the Shock Patient:
Little is usually available to the physician in attendance. Blind administration of IV fluids is not recommended.

For the Cardiopulmonary Arrest Patient:
(1) Basic life support.

(2) If available and patient is apneic, esophageal obturator airway or endotracheal intubation.

(3) Hemodynamic stabilization using AHA-recommended protocol (if equipment and drugs are available). See protocol in Chapter 4.

RISK FACTORS

Identification

While many factors have been shown to increase the risk of developing coronary artery disease, five are primary: serum lipids (primarily cholesterol), smoking, glucose intolerance, systolic blood pressure, and presence of left ventricular hypertrophy (LVH) on ECG. For cholesterol and blood pressure, the risk is a direct and continuous one—that is, it increases without regard for a "normal" value. Age and sex represent two additional important but untreatable factors.

A consideration of each factor as an independent risk in a 50 year old man is illustrated. Data are from the Framingham Study.

Cholesterol. Average value was 236 mg/dl. Risk is doubled when cholesterol increases from 210 to 285.

Smoking. Risk is slightly less than doubled.

Glucose intolerance. Increases risk by approximately one third.

Systolic blood pressure. Average value was 134 mm Hg. Risk is doubled when systolic blood pressure increases from 120 to 180 mm Hg.

LVH on ECG. Risk is doubled.

While each of the factors carries its own risk, the presence of several factors further increases risk. For example, a 50 year old man who does not smoke; has normal glucose tolerance, a cholesterol of 235, and a systolic blood pressure of 135 mm Hg; and does not have LVH on ECG has a risk of developing clinical coronary artery disease of 5% within the next 6 years. The same individual who also smokes has a risk of 8%; if his systolic blood pressure is 180 mm Hg, the risk is increased to 13%; if cholesterol is now 285, risk is increased to 18%; if LVH is present on ECG and glucose intolerance is present, the risk increases to 38%. Risks are therefore additive.

High Density Lipoprotein (HDL) Cholesterol

There is recent evidence that HDL may affect the atherosclerotic process. The relationship is inverse; that is, the higher the HDL, the lower the risk; thus HDL can be considered a "protective" factor. The effect is seen even in the presence of elevations of total cholesterol (or its ultracentrifugation component, low density lipoprotein—LDL cholesterol). Thus the ratio of LDL/HDL may be of more importance than the absolute level of HDL. The mechanism of HDL's effect appears to be related to its function as a transporter of serum lipids to the liver, thus reducing lipid deposition in vascular tissue. Mean HDL cholesterol values for men aged 50–59 have been in the range of 45 mg/dl; in the Framingham Study, risk doubled for each 10 mg/dl *decrease* in HDL cholesterol.

Risk Factor Modification

The association between risk factors and coronary disease is definite; the results of risk factor modification, however, remain controversial. While cholesterol reduction by dietary changes has been associated with decreased risk, a recent trial (Multiple Risk Factor Intervention Trial) has shown nonsignificant improvement in a group having modification of multiple risk factors. Until the question of efficacy of risk factor modification is definitively answered, each physician should be guided by the ease with which the risk factors can be changed and the prevalence and severity of side effects caused by the modification.

REFERENCES

Castelli WP, Doyle JT, Gordon T, et al: HDL cholesterol and other lipids in coronary heart disease: The cooperative lipoprotein phenotyping study. Circulation *55*:767, 1977.

Cobb LA, Wener JA, Trobaugh GE: Sudden cardiac death. I. A decade's experience with out-of-hospital resuscitation. II. Outcome of resuscitation; Management and future direction. Mod Concepts Cardiovasc Dis *49*:31, 1980.

Crampton RS, Aldrich RF, Gascho JA, et al: Reduction of prehospital, ambulance and community coronary death rates by the community-wide emergency cardiac care system. Am J Med *58*:151, 1975.

Dayton S, Pearce ML, Hashimoto, S, et al: A controlled clinical trial of a diet high in unsaturated fat in preventing complication of atherosclerosis. Circulation *40*(Suppl II):1, 1969.

Multiple Risk Factor Intervention Trial: Risk factor changes and mortality results. JAMA *248*:1465, 1982.

II

THE CCU-HOSPITAL PHASE

4

INITIAL HOSPITAL CARE

IN THE EMERGENCY ROOM

General Considerations

Identification

Whether walking or brought by car or ambulance into the Emergency Department, any patient who complains of chest discomfort, nonexertional upper back pain, or epigastric distress should receive immediate evaluation for acute myocardial infarction or myocardial ischemia.

Triage

Can be effectively performed by a nurse or physician's assistant if appropriately trained, as well as by the physician.

Setting

Triage patients should be quickly placed in a room or area in which ACLS-trained personnel are located and which is equipped with cardiac ECG monitor and defibrillator, as well as cardiac emergency drugs and equipment.

If not seen immediately by the physician, continuous ECG monitoring should be instituted and a full 12 lead ECG taken by nursing or technical staff.

Evaluation

Evaluation should be undertaken in two phases—the *initial assessment,* during which a brief search for an immediate life-threatening condition is made, and then a more complete *emergency evaluation.*

Initial Assessment

Each patient, as earlier identified, should be immediately evaluated to determine whether a life-threatening abnormality of vital signs or cardiac rhythm is present, so that prompt treatment can be instituted.

Is blood pressure normal (systolic more than 90 mm Hg or within 30 mm Hg from the patient's normal)? If not, shock or serious hypotension may be present. Systolic pressure less than 90 mm Hg is usually a serious finding in the setting of acute coronary occlusion and, if accompanied by tachycardia or signs of poor perfusion, requires immediate treatment.

Cardiac Rhythm

Is the rhythm regular? If not, is ventricular ectopic activity (requiring immediate drug treatment) present on the monitor? If pulse is greater than 120, is this sinus tachycardia due to anxiety or a reflex response to hypotension and/or cardiac decompensation? Or is it a primary arrhythmia (possibly resulting in hypotension)? If the latter, additional examination and treatment are indicated; this must be done as an emergency if the patient is seriously hypotensive (less than 90 mm Hg systolic).

Respirations

Is the patient short of breath or breathing rapidly? If so, immediate pulmonary examination is necessary to determine whether heart failure or pulmonary edema may be present.

Complete Emergency Assessment

Following the initial, brief examination of vital signs and cardiac rhythm, a complete evaluation should be undertaken. However, this should entail only an examination of pertinent historical, physical, and laboratory findings; the completeness of the examination varies, depending on the findings.

The major objective is to (1) decide whether the patient requires hospital admission, (2) determine whether any immediate diagnostic or therapeutic intervention is necessary, and (3) decide, if appropriate, which area of the hospital is best suited for the patient's care.

Major differential diagnoses to be considered include thoracic aortic dissection, acute pulmonary conditions (including pulmonary embolus, pneumothorax, and pneumonia), mediastinitis, pericarditis, or acute abdominal emergency (such as ruptured peptic ulcer or pancreatitis), as well as acute myocardial infarction.

Additional history suggesting myocardial ischemia includes:

Pain or Discomfort: Variable in nature. Usually retrosternal and oppressive. May extend laterally around chest into either or both shoulders, neck, jaw, and either or both hands. However, may present as upper back or epigastric discomfort. Sharp, shooting, very localized, or tender pain, or pain changing with movement or respirations is not usually characteristic of ischemia or infarction and needs to be thoroughly evaluated.

Associated Symptoms: Shortness of breath (may be indication of left ventricular failure or primary pulmonary disease); nausea, vomiting, urge to defecate; diaphoresis; anxiety.

Response to Nitroglycerin: May be useful in helping evaluate cause of chest discomfort. While relieving ischemic pain, e.g. angina, it may also improve or relieve the pain of acute myocardial infarction and cannot be reliably used by itself to distinguish between these two entities. Relief of discomfort or pain associated with rapid return of ST segment elevation may suggest coronary spasm. Relief is not diagnostic of coronary disease (nitroglycerin is known also to improve or relieve the pain of esophageal spasm).

The ***history*** remains the most important component of the emergency evaluation. Patients with continuous pain compatible with acute myocardial infarction and of more than 30 minutes' duration should be considered to have acute myocardial infarction *even in the absence of physical findings or ECG changes.*

Physical Examination

No abnormalities may be present.

Skin. Cool and diaphoretic. Excessive coolness and diaphoresis are compatible with depression of cardiac output. Cyanosis may be compatible with low cardiac output, right to left shunt, or pulmonary complications.

Pulmonary. Rales in the absence of obstructive lung disease suggest cardiac decompensation. A few posterior basilar rales are usual in the setting of acute myocardial infarction and do not necessarily imply the need for treatment. Wheezing may be a manifestation of pulmonary congestion due to cardiac decompensation, as well as a sign of obstructive lung disease. The lungs in interstitial pulmonary edema may be *normal to auscultation.*

Cardiac. An S4 gallop is frequently seen. Paradoxically split S2 (that is, an S2 in which the two components—aortic and pulmonic—become more widely separated during expiration rather than inspiration) and the presence of an S3 gallop suggest significant left ventricular dysfunction.

Murmur of mitral regurgitation may be compatible with infarction or ischemia of a papillary muscle. Ventricular septal rupture may exist in the early stages of acute myocardial infarction and will have a loud systolic murmur of variable duration at the lower left sternal border. It may be impossible to distinguish murmurs resulting from these two causes on acute physical examination. (See Chapter 22.)

Electrocardiogram

A more complete description will follow. ECG is frequently helpful in substantiating the presence of acute myocardial infarction. It should never be used as a negative finding (i.e., its "normality" should not be interpreted as conclusive evidence that acute myocardial infarction is not present).

Emergency Checklist

This is provided for quick review of all essential components of the emergency evaluation.

When Patient Is Alert:

History

(1) Chest pain/discomfort. Is the chest wall tender? Is it affected by nitroglycerin, respirations, or position?
(2) Diaphoresis?
(3) Nausea, vomiting, hematemesis, melena, jaundice?
(4) Shortness of breath, cough? Hemoptysis?

Physical Findings

(1) Vital signs
(2) Low cardiac output (diaphoresis, cool skin, peripheral cyanosis, depressed mental status)?
(3) Pulses equal in both arms?
(4) Congestive heart failure: neck vein distention, pulmonary rales, gallop rhythms (S3, S4), paradoxically split S2?
(5) Cardiac mechanical disruption: murmur of mitral regurgitation or ventricular septal defect?
(6) Abdomen: enlarged and pulsatile aorta? Femoral pulses similar in nature to brachials?
(7) Edema: extremities or sacral?

Diagnosis and Treatment

(1) Oxygen by mask
(2) ECG
(3) Treatment for pain: If patient is not hypotensive, nitroglycerin, 0.4 mg SL, should be administered. Morphine sulfate is a second-line alternative to nitroglycerin (see Chapter 3)
(4) Chest radiograph:
    (a) To examine the possibility of pulmonary embolus or thoracic aortic aneurysm
    (b) To substantiate suspicion of interstitial pulmonary edema
(5) Arterial blood analysis gas if patient clinically hypoxic, or short of breath, or if pulmonary embolus suspected
(6) IV diuretics if pulmonary edema or severe congestive heart failure is present. Nitroglycerin if moderate congestive heart failure is present
(7) In hypotensive patient, pressor drugs (i.e., levarterenol or dopamine) to maintain systolic blood pressure of 80–90 mm Hg)
(8) Consider transfer: to *Cardiac Catheterization* for hemodynamic instability, suspected acute ventricular septal defect or mitral regurgitation; to *Operating Room* for unstable and rapidly progressive aortic dissection, mitral regurgitation, or ventricular septal defect

When Patient Is Unresponsive:

In the unresponsive or comatose patient, it is essential to recognize the presence of acute myocardial infarction as an associated or related occurrence. Hypotension or hypoxia due to another cause—e.g., blood loss, anaphylactic reaction, drowning—may result in acute myocardial infarction. Remember that severe traumatic injury may result from a loss of consciousness caused by arrhythmia or hypotension in a setting of acute myocardial infarction.

Cardiac Arrest

General Considerations

Standard American Heart Association procedures should be followed. Determination of cardiac rhythm is an important part of the decision making process. Most new defibrillators are equipped with paddles that can also serve as electrodes, allowing the cardiac rhythm to be immediately displayed. This is the preferred approach for immediate ECG review in the cardiac arrest patient, whether arrest occurs in the hospital or before the patient is admitted. "Blind" defibrillation, however, is advocated when prompt determination of the cardiac rhythm is not possible. *Note:* in the following section, energy levels for direct current countershock are in *delivered energy*.

Protocol

Administer Basic Life Support (BLS). If VENTRICULAR FIBRILLATION (VF) IS PRESENT, continue BLS.

Defibrillate at 200–300 joules. If unsuccessful, repeat at the same energy level, continuing BLS during the defibrillator recharging period.

If second countershock is not effective—continue BLS. Assure an effective airway—endotracheal intubation preferred.

Insert IV line.

Give epinephrine, 0.5–1.0 mg IV or via endotracheal route.

Give sodium bicarbonate if arrest longer than 2 minutes prior to effective ventilation. Usual dose: 50–75 ml of solution 1 mEq/ml.

Defibrillate at 360 joules.

If countershock still ineffective, antiarrhythmic drug therapy prior to additional shocks is indicated: lidocaine, 75 mg bolus, or undiluted bretylium, 5 mg/kg bolus.

Additional sodium bicarbonate administration should be determined by specific determination of arterial blood gases.

IF VENTRICULAR TACHYCARDIA IS PRESENT:

Synchronized countershock should be given, with the patient sedated if conscious. An energy level of 20–200 joules is recommended as most effective initially, and may cause less myocardial damage than a full 360 joules.

IF ASYSTOLE IS PRESENT ON INITIAL OR SUBSEQUENT RHYTHM EVALUATIONS:

BLS, effective airway, and IV as above.

Administer epinephrine, 0.5–1.0 mg.

Atropine, 1 mg IV.

If ineffective, calcium chloride, 5 ml of 10% solution.

If asystole continues, additional sodium bicarbonate as dictated by arterial blood gases; epinephrine IV every 5 minutes, and calcium choride every 10 minutes should be given, and IV isoproterenol or intracardiac epinephrine administered.

Dispositon

Patients successfully resuscitated (other than those having a traumatic or metabolic cause for their arrest) should be treated as acute myocardial infarction, despite lack of historical, physical, or electrocardiographic confirmation for infarction; many patients will have a primary arrhythmia as the etiology.

TRANSFER FROM THE EMERGENCY DEPARTMENT

General Considerations

Patients should be treated without delay once myocardial infarction is suspected and other causes are considered as less likely diagnoses. Time in the Emergency Department should be kept at a minimum and the patient transferred to an Intensive or Coronary Care Unit staffed by nurses with CCU training.

Transfer Procedure Checklist

(1) ICU or CCU notified and ready for transfer
(2) Patient comfortable
(3) Continuous ECG monitoring using portable monitor defibrillator
(4) Stable IV in place
(5) Patient has received lidocaine bolus and has appropriate maintenance infusion (see Chapter 3)
(6) Emergency drugs that should accompany patient: (1) lidocaine, 100 mg, (2) atropine, 1 mg, (3) naloxone hydrochloride (Narcan), if large dose of narcotic has been administered
(7) ACLS-trained physician or nurse (this nurse should be certified through the American Heart Association ACLS course; recertification every two years is currently recommended) to accompany patient during transfer
(8) Continuous visual surveillance of patient's general condition and respiration

REFERENCE

Standards and guidelines for cardiopulmonary resuscitation (CPR) and emergency cardiac care (ECC). JAMA *244*:453, 1980.

5

THE CCU ENVIRONMENT, THE PATIENT, AND THE NURSE

*Cynthia A. Padula, M.S., R.N.**

Since its advent in the early 1960s, the Coronary Care Unit (CCU) has undergone tremendous change, as has the entire health care system. Advances in technology over the past two decades have been explosive and a major force behind the growth and evolution of the CCU as we know it today. Computerized arrhythmia monitoring devices, hemodynamic monitoring equipment, and the intraaortic balloon pump illustrate the effect that the technologic boom has had on the nature of cardiovascular medical and nursing practice. Medical research has markedly expanded the theoretical body of knowledge over the past 20 years as well, resulting in unending gains in the diagnosis and treatment of cardiovascular disease. As these advances have evolved, so, too, has the nature of cardiovascular medical and nursing practice.

THE PHYSICAL ENVIRONMENT OF THE CCU

The increasing complexity and sophistication of cardiovascular practice has had profound effects upon the composition and structure of the CCU environment. Likewise, the environment itself clearly has an impact upon all members of the health care team functioning within it.

Ideally, the CCU is geographically distinct from other intensive care units. A quiet, restful environment conducive to optimal stress management is a cornerstone of therapy for the myocardial infarction patient. It is desirable to keep noise levels within the CCU at a minimum to facilitate rest and to prevent possible stress reactions as a result of excessive and unaccustomed sounds.

Each patient room ideally should be designed so the patient can be seen from a central nursing area and should be easily accessible from that point. In considering structural design, it is critically important that the CCU meet the needs of all members of the health care team as well as the needs of the institution. The size of the individual patient rooms, central nurses station, and corridors in particular are also important. Patient rooms should be large enough to allow for easy use of resuscitative equipment, hemody-

*Cardiovascular Clinical Specialist, The Miriam Hospital, Providence, R.I.

namic monitoring equipment, and any of the various other devices routinely utilized. More research is indicated before a conclusive answer can be given to the question of whether single or shared rooms are most therapeutic within the CCU, and for which patients.

Various environmental factors must be considered, including windows for natural lighting; supplemental lighting; colors conducive to relaxation; television sets, telephones, calendars, clocks; assuring patient privacy. In addition, a comfortable family waiting area and private conference room space should be provided, as well as space for medical and nursing conferences.

Within the CCU, the need for an electrically safe environment is readily apparent. It is essential that the critical care nurse maintain an accurate and current knowledge of electrical safety principles. The nurse needs to be skillful in the continuous assessment of the environment for situations and devices that present actual or potential hazards. Periodic inspection of all existing equipment and electrical wiring and the testing of all newly purchased equipment, both performed by a competent engineering staff, are essential.

Another potential hazard to the patient within any CCU is nosocomial infection. Patients in these settings are especially susceptible to infection because of the lowering of normal body defenses associated with illness. This, combined with the frequent use of invasive devices, dramatically increases the potential risk of infection. Infection surveillance and control are essential components within the environment. Every CCU should have policies and procedures specific to infection control. Likewise, education of all team members regarding infection control must be on-going.

THE EMERGENCE OF CARDIOVASCULAR NURSING PRACTICE

Just as the explosion in technology has produced dramatic changes in cardiovascular medicine, so, too, has this evolution changed the nature of nursing. However, these changes have not occurred independently of developments within the profession itself. During the early 1960s, the concept of the nursing process formally emerged as a result of an effort on the part of nursing leaders to define the role of nursing. Nursing process involves the application of problem-solving techniques to the patient care situation. The nursing process is a validation of the unique function of nursing.

The first step of the nursing process involves the nursing assessment. The comprehensive nursing assessment includes such data as history of present illness; past health history; current health status; health beliefs; social, psychologic, cultural, and cognitive assessment; and an assessment of patterns of daily living. Nurses in general, but particularly critical care nurses, have become increasingly competent in utilizing physical assessment skills as an additional means to collect data.

Nursing diagnoses are derived from the assessment of the total patient. Nursing diagnoses are not medical diagnoses; though the nurse works collaboratively with the physician in the treatment of medical problems, the professional nurse develops, implements, and evaluates a nursing plan of care directed at treating identified nursing diagnoses.

The evolution of the cardiovascular nurse illustrates the specialization, redefinition, and emergence of expanded roles that have occurred within nursing. As the focus of CCU interventions evolved to the early recognition and treatment of warning arrhythmias, so also did the role of the nurse dramatically change. With the development of standing drug orders and unit policies allowing for immediate intervention and treatment by the nurse came increased responsibility and independent decision making. Formal educational programs emerged to better prepare CCU nurses for their expanded role. The CCU nurse has rightfully emerged as a competent, knowledgeable professional, an essential member of the health care team.

The scope of cardiovascular nursing practice is not confined to the CCU; it extends to acute, step-down, and rehabilitative focuses as well. Cardiovascular nursing is not institutionally bound, however; nurses in the community, functioning as professional caregivers as well as members of society, are meeting the challenge. The role of the cardiovascular nurse will undoubtedly continue to expand in the future. Technology will continue to advance in leaps and bounds, thus placing increasing demands on the nurse to master and maintain sophisticated technical skills. Meeting the biophysical needs of the critically ill patient requires a nurse who is highly trained in various assessment skills; has a broad knowledge of physiologic principles and clinical application; possesses critical decision-making skills; is an expert in the use of technologic devices; and is able to deliver bedside care of the highest quality. In addition, the nurse must assess and maintain the psychologic integrity of the patient and his or her family, provide an environment conducive to learning, develop a realistic teaching plan, and serve as patient advocate. Nursing in the CCU has become increasingly holistic, individualized, and family-oriented, reflective of an evolving focus within the profession itself.

The development of the clinical specialist role reflects the nursing profession's response to the rapid advances in nursing science and technology. The cardiovascular clinical specialist is a registered nurse with a master's degree in cardiovascular nursing, with an emphasis upon clinical practice. The clinical nurse specialist is an expert clinician who functions in the role of educator, consultant, and researcher. The clinical specialist possesses expert power derived from advanced clinical knowledge and serves as a role model and a change agent with the institution.

Cardiovascular nursing, though in its infancy, has developed into a distinct entity within the nursing profession. Advances in cardiovascular medicine and nursing are certain to alter dramatically the course of health care; cardiovascular nurses, as professionals and consumers, will continue to lead the way toward cardiovascular health.

EFFECT OF THE CCU ENVIRONMENT ON THE PATIENT

Psychologic safety is a fundamental need of all individuals. The literature reflects the growing concerns about the psychologic problems experienced by Critical Care Unit patients. However, after interviewing 100 patients, Cassem, Hackett, Bascom, and Wishnie (1970) concluded that the patient in the CCU reacts very differently to the environment than do patients within other ICUs. In addition, they noted that little attention had been given to the potential of the CCU environment actually to alleviate anxiety of patients. An additional major conclusion was that the nurse was the member of the health team most able to alleviate anxiety effectively.

Hackett and Cassem (1975) noted that patients suffering from a myocardial infarction experience a sequence of behavioral reactions: anxiety, peaking during the first 48 hours; denial, which appears around day 2 and normally dissipates by the third or fourth day; and depression, usually seen from the third to the sixth day.

It is vital that patients in the CCU be allowed and encouraged to express their anxieties, fears, and concerns if and when they choose; it is essential to remember, however, that not all patients will exhibit this behavior. Using the nursing process, the CCU nurse assesses the patient's health belief model, coping history, and ability to employ successful coping strategies in the illness. In addition, the nurse continually assesses the environment, the patient's psychologic response to it, and the response to illness. An atmosphere of trust is essential and is most likely to develop when the patient views the nurse as competent, readily available, and supportive of both physical and psychologic needs. The nurse must continually assess and manipulate the environment to assure that it is conducive to optimal rest and recovery and is indeed therapeutic.

Hoffman, Donckers, and Hauser (1978) conducted a study designed to assist nurses to intervene in and reduce stress perceived by patients in a CCU. Factors identified as most stressful by patients included the illness itself; visiting regulations; bedrest; sleep interruptions; loss of privacy; and noise level in the unit. The researchers concluded that nurses skilled in the identification and management of stressors in the environment are effective in reducing patient stress.

Teaching has been demonstrated to decrease anxiety levels. Teaching must be individualized to meet individual patient needs and requires continual assessment of teaching and learning needs. Developing a trusting relationship is critically important in providing an environment conducive to learning. Much of the teaching that takes place in the CCU, particularly initially, focuses on orientation to the environment and its components. Such teaching is designed to achieve the short-term goal of stress reduction. Inadequate patient education serves to foster anxiety, emotional stress, and inadequate coping.

There is general agreement that explanatory patient education concerning the environment should begin immediately upon admission into the CCU. The literature indicates disagreement, however, as to whether formal teaching should begin in the CCU or not. It is essential that the nurse assess each patient and family individually for learning needs and emotional and intellectual readiness to learn. In this manner, teaching is based upon realistic patient needs and is not a rigid, inflexible collection of program objectives designed to meet the needs of the health care providers.

Transitional teaching is essential in order to prepare the patient and family for transfer from the CCU. Transfer represents a concrete sign of improvement but is not without accompanying anxieties and concerns. Minckley et al (1979) state that transfer without adequate preparation may induce the stress response, which can precipitate chest pain and arrhythmias in addition to fear, anger, and anxiety.

Unfortunately, patients are often transferred quickly with no preparation because of poor planning, failure to recognize the need for transfer preparation, or a realistic demand for beds. The CCU nurse plays a major role in identifying the need for transfer preparation and in providing the teaching needed. The nurse also assesses the patient's and family's responses to instruction and continues to provide a supportive environment during the transfer process. Likewise, nurses on the transfer unit must continue to reinforce patient understanding, assess negative effects of transfer, and intervene appropriately.

EFFECT OF THE CCU ENVIRONMENT ON THE FAMILY

Little has been written about the effects of the CCU environment upon the family of the critically ill patient. A holistic approach to nursing requires that the patient be viewed as a biophysical, psychosocial being, who functions as a member of a family system.

Within the CCU environment, where patient survival is often the foremost priority, identification and satisfaction of family needs often become secondary. The family's response to illness may include fear, helplessness, shock, disbelief, guilt, loneliness, and depression. The complexity of the CCU itself is likely to increase anxiety and fear, particularly if family members are totally unfamiliar with the environment. The development of a trusting relationship with the family as soon as possible after the patient is admitted to the CCU is essential. Open channels of communication between family members and members of the health care team are crucially important; providing the family with accurate, on-going, and current information serves to decrease anxiety. It is important to encourage families to address their concerns and express their feelings with staff members; likewise, nursing staff must attempt to facilitate a conducive environment in which interaction with family members is considered to be a priority. The nurse continually assesses the stressors affecting family members, as well as their reactions to them, and develops strategies for intervention. Identifying with family members the essential role that they play in their loved one's recovery and incorporating them into decision making and various aspects of care benefits all members of the team. The healthy family, when fully utilized, serves as an invaluable provider of information concerning the patient, as well as support during the illness and recovery period.

EFFECT OF THE CCU ENVIRONMENT ON THE NURSE

The reality of day-to-day encounters with critical illness, its manifestations, and its implications all place great stresses upon the nurse. The ever-expanding roles and responsibilities of the CCU nurse have provided sources of stress within the environment, as have multiple other developments in health care. In a highly technologic environment in which the threat of death is ever present, it becomes easy, and indeed is sometimes a relief, for the nurse to focus on the physical and technical aspects of illness alone. Unfortunately, little emphasis in the past has been placed on assisting nurses to cope with stress in an attempt to prevent total depletion of their coping reserve. Support systems must be present, highly utilized, and accepted as critically important within the environment. The current literature reflects increasing application of this concept in CCUs.

CCU nursing staff deal continually with the patient's response to illness, which may be manifested in a variety of ways. Each behavior is a cue to the presence of an underlying need and requires the nurse to be sensitive to those needs. Such situations, though they have the potential to be extremely rewarding, can also be emotionally draining, particularly when combined with the other realistic, multiple stresses and conflicts of critical care nursing. Likewise, assisting the families of critically ill patients through the illness experience, though identified and accepted as an essential role of nursing, frequently generates a significant amount of stress.

Dealing with death is a common experience in the CCU and likewise is a realistic source of stress. Death may precipitate feelings of failure, guilt, depression, denial, and anger in nursing staff. Repeated exposure to these reactions without the achievement of acceptance and resolution can lead to emotional detachment and withdrawal. Repeated attachments and losses may facilitate the development of group pessimisim or depression (Eisendrath and Dunkel, 1979).

The CCU presents an array of ethical dilemmas that all members of the health care team must deal with on a daily basis. Often the conflicts that arise focus on issues of maintaining quality of life versus preservation of life.

Support of the need for a collaborative physician-nurse relationship within the health care system has been growing. However, it is also evident that nurses and physicians within the CCU setting often find themselves in conflict. The origin of these conflicts often revolves around ethical issues, clinical decision making, and communication. Allen, Jackson, and Younger (1980) suggest that the disagreements may arise from the nurse's perception of noninvolvement in decision making; they suggest joint sessions to deal openly with conflicts, as well as clearer delineation of professional goals. The unavailability of physicians in times of need is another source of conflict frequently identified by nurses.

Interpersonal conflicts between nurses themselves have been reported as a source of stress. The nature of the CCU environment demands cooperation, mutual respect, open communication, and on-going but often crisis-oriented support. Maladaptive group behavior, if not effectively identified and treated, can lead to a deterioration of group morale, which can negatively affect the quality of patient care. The value of a support group to assist nurses, both as individuals and as members of a group, to deal with the stresses associated with CCU nursing cannot be overstated.

Excessive workloads resulting from inadequate staffing is a frequently cited source of conflict for the nurse. Additionally, a lack of understanding on the part of nursing administrators in regard to the demands of CCU nursing is often identified by the staff nurse. Again, mutual respect and understanding and the maintenance of open lines of communication are essential. The therapeutic group setting often can offer the support and understanding necessary to assist nursing staff to meet the challenges of critical care nursing.

One might be led to ask the question: Why choose coronary care nursing at all? As stated so clearly by Cassem, Nelson, and Rich (1979), "Paradoxically, the source of the greatest stress and of the greatest satisfaction is the same: caring for desperately ill patients. It is at once the hazard and the honor of the coronary care unit nurse."

REFERENCES

Allen M, Jackson D, Younger S: Closing the communication gap between physicians and nurses in the intensive care unit setting. Heart Lung *9*:836, 1980.

Cassem NH, Hackett TP, Bascom C, Wishnie H: Reactions of coronary patients to the CCU nurse. Am J Nurs *70*:320, 1970.

Cassem NH, Nelson K, Rich RR: The nurse in the coronary care unit, *in* Gentry WD, Williams RB Jr (eds): Psychological Aspects of Myocardial Infarction and Coronary Care. 2nd ed. St. Louis, C. V. Mosby, 1979.

Eisendrath S J, Dunkel J: Psychological issues in the intensive care unit staff. Heart Lung *8*:751, 1979.

Hackett TP, Cassem NH: Coronary Care: Patient Psychology. New York, American Heart Association, 1975.

Hoffman M, Donckers S, Hauser M: The effect of nursing interventions on stress factors perceived by patients in a coronary patient unit. Heart Lung *7*:804, 1978.

Minckley B, Burrows D, Ehrat K, et al: Myocardial infarction stress-of-transfer inventory: Development of a research tool. Nurs Res *28*:4, 1979.

SUGGESTED READING

Caldwell T, Weiner M: Stresses and coping in intensive care nursing. I. A review. Gen Hosp Psychiatr *3*:119, 1981.

Hackett TP, Cassem NH, Wishnie H: Detection and treatment of anxiety in the coronary care unit. Am Heart J *78*:727, 1969.

Molter NC: Needs of relatives of critically ill patients: A descriptive study. Heart Lung *8*:332, 1979.

Murphy CP: The moral situation in nursing, *in* Bandam E, Bandam P: Bioethics and Human Rights: A Reader for Health Professionals. Boston, Little, Brown, and Company, 1978.

Toth JC: Effects of structured preparation for transfer on patient anxiety on leaving coronary care unit. Nurs Res *29*:28, 1980.

6

CCU ORDERS

Many different therapeutic approaches to the management of patients with suspected myocardial infarction are available, and aspects of the pharmacologic and mechanical interventions that may be employed during the acute phase of myocardial ischemia will be discussed in depth in succeeding chapters. However, prior to any discussion of *specific* therapeutic/management alternatives, it seems appropriate to designate a set of admission orders comprising a systematic checklist of monitoring, activities, diet, medications, diagnostic laboratory tests, and ancillary studies that should be implemented for the patient admitted to the Coronary Care Unit (CCU) with a suspected myocardial infarction (MI).

It is acknowledged that there are many formats or programs that are not only appropriate but also medically sound, for use as admission orders to the CCU. Such "standing orders" have been employed with success in CCUs but are often regarded as rigid, inflexible, and occasionally offensive to many physicians and nurses, who rightly view them as being too arbitrary and generalized for individual patients. However, it appears that this criticism centers primarily on the *content* of a proposed set of admission orders, not on the *concept* that such an approach would be a desirable one.

The regimen given here offers a systematic checklist of orders that afford comprehensive, yet flexible, guidelines for patients admitted to a CCU. The purpose of these orders is to ensure that several important categories for diagnostic and therapeutic recommendations are covered, and that the physician can be allowed to exercise the flexibility of choice for any given patient. Above all, these suggested guidelines, which may be found on pages 34–35, embody a means of minimizing errors of omission, or oversights, when a patient is admitted to the CCU.

The purposes of the specific CCU orders are briefly described:

1. ADMIT. The patient's name and medical service/attending physician are listed here.
2. DIAGNOSIS. In general, a specific diagnosis should be recorded—e.g., acute inferior MI, anterior wall MI with pulmonary edema. Frequently the phrase "rule out (R/O) MI" is used on this line.
3. CONDITION. Most patients with evolving myocardial infarction or R/O myocardial infarction are considered in serious or critical condition.
4. ALLERGIES. It is important that allergies to medication be listed specifically in the order sheet. Preferably, a notation of a

specific drug allergy is taped on the front of the patient's chart and/or noted over the patient's bed.

5. MONITORING. All patients should be placed on continuous cardiac monitoring for the purpose of recording abnormalities of rate and rhythm.

The physician or house officer should be notified of any changes in rhythm or rate, particularly the development of ventricular ectopic activity—that is, PVCs, couplets, multiform PVCs, and so on.

Vital signs vary among CCUs. In general, most Coronary Care Units utilize a standard regimen like this: Vital signs q 30 min × 4; q 60 min × 2; if stable, q 2 hr throughout the initial 24 hr; q 4 hr thereafter. If such is the case, CCU routine is checked under "Vital sign" orders. Any other specific changes from the usual regimen are listed specifically under "other."

Specific intake and output (hourly and every shift) are extremely important to quantify, particularly for the patient in congestive heart failure in whom very specific information is needed to assess the response to dietary manipulations and diuretic usage.

Swan-Ganz measurements are listed to include a recording of pulmonary arterial (PA) pressures and pulmonary capillary wedge (PCW) pressures. In patients who are invasively monitored for myocardial infarction or complications arising therefrom, PA pressures should be recorded at least every 30–60 minutes. Depending on the clinical instability of the patient, PCW pressures likewise may be recorded as frequently as PA pressures, although the risk of inadvertent "overwedging" of the balloon-tipped catheter (or the permanent "wedging" of the PA catheter in the distal pulmonary arterial capillary bed) increases as a function of the frequency that these latter measurements are obtained. (See also Chapter 12.)

Where there is good correlation between pulmonary artery end-diastolic pressure (PAEDP) and PCW pressure, we prefer to use the PAEDP to guide the ongoing assessment of left ventricular filling pressure and changes in therapy that are needed. In general, PCW determinations are often needed only once or twice per shift.

Intra-arterial blood pressure (BP) measurements likewise are recorded in either the phasic or mean pressure modality. In the case of both Swan-Ganz and intra-arterial pressure measurements, the physician or house officer should be notified if there are changes in these parameters, which is designated as follows: Notify house officer if systolic BP decreases below 90 mm Hg; notify house officer if PCW pressure increases above 18 mm Hg, and so on.

Respirator settings, if the patient is intubated and on assisted ventilation, are listed to include the inspired oxygen concentration (FIO_2), tidal volume (TV), respiratory rate (rate), and so on.

Most patients who are admitted to the CCU without pulmonary edema or respiratory failure are managed with supplemental oxygen via nasal cannula. The concentration of oxygen generally ranges

1. ADMIT ______________ SERVICE __________
2. DIAGNOSIS:
3. CONDITION: Satisfactory Serious Critical
4. ALLERGIES:
5. MONITORING:
   - ______ Cardiac monitor
   - ______ Notify house officer for PVCs
   - ______ Vital signs
     - ______ CCU routine
     - ______ Other ______________
   - ______ Intake & output ______ q shift; ______ hourly
   - ______ Swan-Ganz measurements (if applicable):
     - ______ PA pressures, PCW q ______
     - ______ notify house officer if ______________
   - ______ Intra-arterial BP (if applicable):
     - ______ phasic; ______ mean pressures q ______
     - ______ notify house officer if ______________
   - ______ Respirator settings (if applicable):
     - ______ FIO_2;______TV;______rate;______mode
   - ______ Oxygen ______ L/min; ______ other __________
6. ACTIVITY:
   - ______ Strict bed rest
   - ______ Bedrest & commode (Level I)
   - ______ Bed/chair/commode (Level II)
   - ______ Bed/chair/bathroom/walk in room (Level III)
   - ______ Other ______________
7. DIET:
   - ______ Cardiac diet, frequent small meals
   - ______ ADA diet
   - ______ 90 mEq Na^+ (2 gm Na^+)
   - ______ Other ______________
8. MEDICATIONS:
   - ______ Analgesic ______________
   - ______ Antiarrhythmic ______________
     ____
   - ______ Propranolol ______________
   - ______ Digoxin ______________
   - ______ Diuretic ______________

Continued on opposite page

_____ NTG _____
_____ Anticoagulant _____
_____ Tranquilizer _____
_____ Sleeping medication _____
_____ Stool softener _____
_____
_____
_____

9. IV ORDERS:
   _____ D_5W KVO
   _____ _____
   _____ _____
   _____
   _____

10. LABORATORY TESTS:
    _____ Stat portable CXR, if not done in ER; then daily
    _____ Daily ECG; _____ ECG during any chest pain
    _____ Cardiac enzymes
        _____ **If MI suspected,** CPK enzymes (including isoenzymes) at 8, 16, 24 hours p admission; LDH, SGOT, SGPT qd × 2 days
        _____ other _____
    _____ Chemistry profile (SMA 7 or 12)
    _____ Lipid profile (fasting serum cholesterol, triglyceride, and HDL-cholesterol), if less than 24 hr from the onset of symptoms
    _____ CBC, PTA, PTT, platelet estimate
    _____ Urinalysis
    _____ Other _____
    _____
    _____

11. ANCILLARY ITEMS:
    _____ Weigh daily; _____ qod
    _____ Elastic stockings
    _____ Footboard
    _____ Passive and active leg and arm exercises
    _____ Cardiac teaching post-MI
    _____ Other _____

12. MD'S SIGNATURE _____

from 2 to 5 L/min and should be so recorded on the order sheet. Occasionally, higher inspired flow concentrations or controlled oxygen delivery with the use of the Venturi mask is indicated. These specific usages are so recorded.

6. ACTIVITY. In general, patients are relegated to strict bedrest or to bedrest and commode (Level I) during the first 24 hours of hospitalization in the CCU. In uncomplicated MIs during the second day or in patients in whom MIs have been excluded, activity may be appropriately liberalized to Levels II or III as noted.

7. DIET. Diet is discussed in detail in Chapter 7. In general, a cardiac diet consisting of frequent small meals and one that is low in cholesterol, low in saturated fat, and soft in bulk is preferred. When rigid sodium restriction is not necessary, no added salt (NAS), equivalent to approximately 6 grams of sodium, is a reasonable alternative.

8. MEDICATIONS. These are discussed in considerable detail in Chapters 16 and 17.

Analgesics: Morphine sulfate or meperidine (Demerol) is a useful analgesic agent often used in the setting of acute myocardial infarction. Morphine sulfate in incremental IV doses ranging between 2 and 5 mg every 5 to 15 min (to a total dose not to exceed 20 mg) is a useful regimen. Meperidine (25–50 mg) can be given slowly via the intravenous route, but care should be taken to observe any changes in BP or heart rate. Occasionally, oral agents such as hydromorphone (Dilaudid) are preferred by some physicians for the relief of ischemic cardiac pain.

Repeated doses of analgesics should be given at regular intervals for pain relief.

Antiarrhythmic: In general, lidocaine is the drug of choice and should be administered to all patients who display evidence of ventricular ectopic activity complicating suspected infarction. See Chapter 3 for prophylactic usage and Chapter 15 for standard antiarrhythmic usage.

Propranolol, digoxin, diuretic, nitroglycerin, anticoagulants: Patients on any or all of these medications should be continued on these agents unless there is a specific indication for discontinuing their usage. Examples of this are withholding digoxin in suspected digoxin toxicity and discontinuing (or tapering) beta-blockers such as propranolol in a patient with myocardial infarction, if it is complicated by congestive heart failure.

Tranquilizer: Psychologic factors are known to contribute to the genesis of pain, ischemia, and frequently to arrhythmias. Many patients will respond favorably to doses of diazepam (Valium), 5–10 mg q 6 hr. Alternatively, chlordiazepoxide (Librium), in a dose of 10 mg q 6 hr, or oxazepam (Serax), 10–15 mg po q 4–6 hr, may be employed.

Sleeping medication: Flurazepam (Dalmane), 15–30 mg, is frequently employed as a sleeping medication. This drug has a minimal effect on disturbing REM sleep patterns and is well tolerated by most cardiac patients.

Stool softener: Dioctyl sodium sulfosuccinate (Colace), 100 mg po qd is a safe and effective stool softener. In constipation, milk of magnesia, 30 ml po hs prn is administered for intermittent laxative use.

9. IV ORDERS. Many uncomplicated MI patients or "rule out MI" patients will receive only a dextrose and water infusion at the minimum infusion rate (D5W KVO). Other intravenous fluid orders, such as isotonic (normal) saline or combinations of saline and dextrose, are specified with a per hour infusion rate, including any supplements such as potassium chloride.

10. LABORATORY TESTS. All patients should have an admission chest radiograph (CXR) prior to, or shortly after, admission to the CCU.

Serial ECGs on a daily basis are necessary to observe sequential changes in patients admitted with suspected infarction. It is imperative to obtain ECGs during episodes of chest pain for the purpose of comparing these ischemic changes to other baseline ECGs.

Cardiac enzyme determinations should be obtained in all patients with suspected infarction, and at least four CPK enzyme levels (including isoenzymes) should be obtained at 6–8 hr intervals after admission to the hospital. More frequent sampling may be necessary in patients with ongoing ischemia.

Other enzyme measurements (LDH, SGOT) should be obtained daily for 2–3 days. (See Chapter 8.)

Routine blood determinations, including a chemistry profile, complete blood count, and urinalysis should be obtained on admission and on a daily or every-other-day basis. More frequent sampling of serum sodium and potassium levels may be required, particularly in patients on incremental diuretic therapy.

The fasting lipid profile is of particular concern, since reliable data may be obtained for baseline cholesterol, triglyceride, and HDL cholesterol values within the first 24 hours after admission. Thereafter, changes in lipids and lipoproteins induced by myocardial infarction and/or hospitalization may adversely affect these parameters.

11. ANCILLARY ITEMS. Daily weights, elastic stockings, footboard, and passive and active leg and arm exercises are all desirable interventions for the bedridden patient in the CCU.

7
CCU DIET AND ACTIVITY

DIET

General Considerations

Few scientific studies guide diet selection for the patient who is admitted to the Coronary Care Unit (CCU) with suspected myocardial infarction (MI). In general, patients are kept NPO or on clear liquids during the first 12–24 hours after admission, and fluid intake (combined IV and oral) in the uncomplicated MI patient is limited to between 1500–2500 ml in order to maintain an adequate urinary output (800–1200 ml). The rationale for this approach is as follows:

1. Meals containing solid food may precipitate angina pectoris and can contribute to increased myocardial oxygen demand in patients with acute ischemic heart disease;
2. Many patients become nauseated—as a result of anxiety, narcotic analgesic administration, or following acute inferior wall myocardial infarction characterized often by elevated parasympathomimetic activity—and will be unable to ingest solid food;
3. The risk of aspiration is minimized if solid food is avoided during the initial 12–24 hours of hospitalization. Electrical complications of myocardial infarction (cardiac arrest, ventricular fibrillation, and so on) occur in a finite percentage of acute MI patients in the first 24 hours of admission to the CCU, and aspiration of solid contents may result during defibrillation or resuscitation.

After the first 12–24 hours (or when the patient becomes pain-free without evidence of continuing ischemia), diet is advanced to a soft, low sodium, low cholesterol diet. Ideally, meals should be small in quantity and spaced at frequent intervals (4–6/day), to prevent indigestion and any unwanted postprandial increases in cardiac output, which may occur after heavy meals. In the MI patient with complications (individuals with persistent pain, arrhythmias, congestive heart failure, invasive hemodynamic monitoring), oral intake may have to be limited to fluids alone for longer time periods, and an intravenous infusion of either 5% glucose or glucose in saline may have to be maintained until the patient stabilizes.

Patients with impaired left ventricular function (due to acute myocardial necrosis or secondary to chronic ischemic heart disease) and depressed cardiac output may exhibit sodium retention. Thus, the liberal use of dietary sodium should be discouraged in the CCU, since pulmonary congestion and/or hypervolemia may supervene. In contrast, rigid sodium restriction—especially in patients with a "borderline" systemic arterial pressure (90–100 mm Hg) and clear lung fields—may result in hypovolemia with ensuing aggravation of low blood pressure, cardiac output, and urinary output.

Therefore, in uncomplicated MI patients (or patients admitted to the CCU with suspected infarction), a no-added-salt (4–5 gm NaCl/24 hr) regimen may be satisfactory, while in patients with evident hypervolemia (CHF), more rigid dietary sodium restriction is warranted.

It has been the practice in many CCUs to proscribe the use of hot or cold beverages, on the assumption that they may precipitate arrhythmias or conduction disturbances. However, more recent data do not support this contention, and patients can safely ingest hot or cold fluids as desired.

The use of caffeine-rich beverages (coffee, tea, cola) should be avoided in patients admitted to the CCU because of the positive inotropic and chronotropic effects of methylated xanthines and their possible arrhythmogenic effects. Decaffeinated coffee, tea, or cola may be permitted with meals.

Patients with ischemic heart disease may require dietary counseling and, in some cases, reeducation. Many individuals with acute myocardial infarction display a simplistic, often unrealistic, knowledge about the role of dietary cholesterol and saturated fats in the development of their ischemic event. While the role of dietary cholesterol in the pathogenesis of myocardial infarction remains controversial, most physicians feel that dietary modification to a low cholesterol, low saturated fat intake (e.g., limited ingestion of eggs, animal fats, butter, cream) with a proportionately increased amount of polyunsaturated fat intake is a commonsense approach. Some patients mistakenly believe that modification of saturated fat intake in middle or late life may prevent or reverse coronary atherosclerosis.

Clearly, the CCU provides an ideal initial environment for such dietary reeducation, and the services of a good dietitian are extremely important to facilitate patient instruction and behavior modification. Again, strict scientific data are not available to guide prospective diet therapy, although measurement of a fasting lipid profile and the assessment of ideal body weight are important in determining which individuals may benefit most from dietary modification. Obviously, consideration must be given to the age and weight of the patient, history of previous MI, and the severity of illness. For example, rigid dietary cholesterol restriction would seem ill-advised in an elderly patient who is not overweight and whose lipid profile is normal.

It has been customary to defer measurement of serum cholesterol and triglycerides in the acute infarct patient until later in convalescence, since acute changes in lipids and lipoproteins have been reported in the acute phase of myocardial infarction. Recent studies indicate, however, that the reductions in cholesterol and HDL-cholesterol are not manifest until 36–48 hours after infarction. These studies indicate that a fasting lipid profile obtained on admission (or on the morning after admission) appears to correlate well with baseline values 8–12 weeks after infarction. Thus, it is appropriate to assess a patient's lipid status soon after admission and adjust the subsequent diet accordingly.

Finally, glucose-insulin-potassium (GIK) infusions have been advocated by some investigators as a useful adjunct in the management of acute myocardial infarction (the Sodi-Pallares "polarizing treatment" for acute myocardial infarction). This consisted of infusion of 10% glucose solution with 40 mEq of potassium chloride/L and 20 units of insulin/L at a rate of 40–60 drops per minute. Since this initial report in 1960, several conflicting studies have been reported regarding the purported efficacy of GIK infusions in preventing arrhythmias and limiting infarct size. Recent clinical trials indicate that there is a reduction in mortality in patients treated with this solution, but, to date, there is little conclusive evidence from which to advocate the widespread use of GIK infusions in the CCU.

Recommendations

In Uncomplicated Myocardial Infarction:

NPO for the first 12–24 hours; except, if the patient is pain-free and without symptoms of respiratory compromise, clear liquids may be used for the initial 12–24 hours after admission to the CCU.

Advance on second day to soft, no-added-salt, low cholesterol, low saturated fat diet in multiple (4–6) small portions.

Hot or cold beverages, decaffeinated beverages as desired.

No tobacco products.

Fasting lipid profile (serum cholesterol, HDL-cholesterol, and triglycerides) within one day of admission to the CCU.

In Complicated Myocardial Infarction:

NPO until pain-free or hemodynamically stable (generally, first 24 hours).

Intravenous fluids (5% glucose in water, glucose in saline, isotonic saline, etc.) as needed to maintain adequate systemic arterial pressure, urine output, and, if indicated, left ventricular filling pressure (see Chapters 16, 17, 19).

Initiate oral feedings and advance diet on an individual basis, according to the patient's clinical status.

In patients with congestive heart failure, sodium intake should be more rigidly restricted; e.g., 0.5–2.0 grams Na^+ per day, according to clinical situation.

Fasting lipid profile (serum cholesterol, HDL-cholesterol, and triglycerides) within one day of admission to the CCU.

BEDREST/ACTIVITY

General Considerations

During the last decade, the approach to in-hospital activity of the coronary patient has evolved toward early ambulation and discharge. Until the late 1940s, protracted bedrest and hospitalization were the cornerstone of treatment for myocardial infarction. This was predicated on pathologic studies of the healing process following myocardial infarction, which affirmed the concept that at least 6 weeks were required for transformation of necrotic myocardium to firm scar tissue; this fostered the empiric belief that any physical exertion would markedly increase the occurrence of ventricular aneurysm or rupture, arrhythmia, recurrent infarction, or sudden death.

Gradually, these concepts were outmoded over the ensuing half-century; most clinicians now feel that early ambulation for appropriately selected patients after uncomplicated myocardial infarction is no longer controversial. However, as recently as the early 1970s, there was a remarkable heterogeneity in physician attitudes toward activity after myocardial infarction, with the duration of bedrest varying from 1 day to 4 weeks after uncomplicated infarction and the duration of hospitalization ranging from 2–6 weeks. It is now generally acknowledged that most serious complications and fatalities from myocardial infarction occur during the first few days of hospitalization and that the overwhelming majority of uncomplicated infarct patients have little or no in-hospital mortality and extremely few significant complications.

Several adverse physiologic and pathologic effects occur with prolonged immobilization at bedrest: a decrease in physical work capacity, loss of normal postural vasomotor reflexes, increased risk of significant thromboembolism, a modest decrease in pulmonary ventilation caused by depression of lung volume and vital capacity at bedrest, negative nitrogen and protein balances, and, perhaps most important, decreases in skeletal muscle mass and muscular contractile strength and efficiency. Thus, the benefits of early ambulation appear to center on the prevention of physical deconditioning and the other pathophysiologic sequelae of prolonged bedrest. In addition, early ambulation postinfarction may prevent or ameliorate anxiety and depression and may facilitate a greater physical capacity at discharge.

Most acute MI patients at present stay in the CCU 2–4 days and in the hospital 10–21 days. Some investigators have shown that as many as 50% of patients with confirmed myocardial infarction admitted to the CCU can be discharged safely at 7 days, but this remains controversial. Recently, Roberts and coworkers reported that the incidence of in-hospital reinfarction following initial *non-transmural* infarction may be as high as 40%, occurring 10–14 days after hospitalization. Thus, there is a scientific basis for the emerging conservative trend of hospitalizing patients for a full 2 weeks—even following an "uncomplicated" infarction.

In many institutions, telemetry units, or "stepdown" units, provide a comprehensive level of intermediate coronary care; these special facilities may embody a computerized arrhythmia surveillance system in a "dedicated" cardiovascular unit with skilled nursing personnel and other health care professionals (see Chapter 26).

Recommendations

Coronary Care Unit

In general, ambulation is guided by the patient's condition, including both subjective and objective signs that myocardial ischemia has abated. In *uncomplicated* myocardial infarction, most patients are admitted and kept in the CCU for 2 to 4 days, or for at least 48 hours following their last major complication (serious ventricular ectopy, chest pain, congestive heart failure [CHF], etc.). Several protocols have been developed for activity levels in the CCU. A simple scheme is presented here:

Strict bedrest (Level I)
Bedrest with commode privileges (Level II)
Bed/chair/commode (Level III)
Bed/chair/bathroom; may walk in room (Level IV)

By definition, a *complicated* MI patient (persistent chest pain, CHF, arrhythmias, invasive monitoring) would most likely be maintained at Level I, although occasionally at Level II, assuming that the upright position does not result in deterioration of stable hemodynamics. In contrast, an *uncomplicated* MI patient might be admitted with Level II activity and, if stable, be advanced to Level III on day 2 or 3 in the CCU. It would be rare to achieve Level IV activity in the CCU under most circumstances involving acute myocardial ischemia/infarction.

During Level I activity, the patient may use a footboard, and passive range of motion exercises may be commenced on day 2. Antiembolic stockings are applied, and they are removed for 30 minutes every nursing shift. In the absence of chest pain, severe CHF, cardiogenic shock, serious ventricular arrhythmias, or high-grade atrioventricular (AV) block, the patient is advanced to Level III on day 2. The duration of time out of bed increases in a stepwise fashion and depends on the development of fatigue or complications such as angina, arrhythmias, marked tachycardia, or postural hypertension.

For the uncomplicated MI patient, such activities as feeding oneself, washing hands and face, and brushing teeth are permitted on day 2, while shaving, a complete bedbath, and hair combing are generally initiated on day 3.

Telemetry Unit and/or Medical Ward

Uncomplicated MI patients are generally transferred to the Intermediate Care Unit or general medical ward between days 2 and 4 following admission to the CCU. Unless complications supervene, their activity is advanced to Level IV by day 4, with assistance to the bathroom. By days 5–6, they are permitted to walk to the bathroom and begin limited walking in the room. Between days 6–10, the patient is permitted to take short walks on the ward, at first with assistance. From day 9 to discharge, the patient is allowed to gradually increase ambulation as tolerated. These guidelines are flexible and are predicated on the fact that no complications ensue after admission. In general, patients with uncomplicated transmural infarctions are discharged 14–21 days after admission, and patients with uncomplicated nontransmural infarctions are discharged in 12–14 days (see preceding section, under General Considerations).

OTHER ACTIVITIES

Smoking. The use of tobacco products in the CCU is strictly prohibited. The acute circulatory effects of cigarette smoking involve excessive endogenous catecholamine release, increased heart rate (and myocardial oxygen consumption), and possible release of vasoactive substances (prostaglandin endoperoxides, thromboxane A_2), which may produce potent vasoconstrictor and platelet aggregator effects.

The *emotional impact* of acute myocardial infarction and of the hospitalization in the CCU may be extremely anxiety provoking. A deliberate effort should be made to maintain the atmosphere in the CCU as quiet and restful as is practical. Attempts to offset apprehension by careful explanations of the nature of the illness should be made. The role and purpose of equipment and procedures should be thoroughly explained. Because patients may have a difficult time adjusting to this "intensive" environment, and since a high percentage of individuals who were cigarette smokers may experience increased agitation from nicotine withdrawal, mild sedation with oxazepam (10–15 mg q 4–6 hr) or diazepam (2–5 mg q 4–6 hr) is routinely employed to allay anxiety. (See Chapter 6.)

Exercise testing post–MI. See Chapter 26.

SUGGESTED READING

Burch GE: Sick people's food. Am Heart J *85*:279, 1973.

Cohen IM, Alpert JS, Francis GS, et al: Safety of hot and cold liquids in patients with acute myocardial infarction. Chest *71*:450, 1977.

Doyle JT: Tobacco and the cardiovascular system, *In* Hurst JW: The Heart. 4th ed. New York, McGraw-Hill, 1978.

Fyfe T, Baxter RH, Cochran KM, et al: Plasma lipid changes after myocardial infarction. Lancet *2*:997, 1971.

Hutter AM Jr, DeSanctis RW, Flynn T, et al: Non-transmural myocardial infarction: A comparison of hospital and late clinical course of patients with that of matched patients with transmural anterior and transmural inferior myocardial infarction. Am J Cardiol *48*:595, 1981.

Inside the Coronary Care Unit. A guide for the patient and family. Pamphlet, American Heart Association, Dallas.

Marmor A, Sobel BE, Roberts R: Factors presaging early recurrent myocardial infarction ("extension"). Am J Cardiol *48*:603, 1981.

McNeer JF, Wagner GS, Ginsburg PB, et al: Hospital discharge one week after acute myocardial infarction. N Engl J Med *298*:229, 1978.

Ritchie JM: Central nervous system stimulants. II. The xanthines, *In* Goodman LS, Gilman A (eds): The Pharmacologic Basis of Therapeutics. 3rd ed. New York, The Macmillan Company, 1965.

Wenger NK, Hellerstein HK: Rehabilitation of the Coronary Patient. New York, John Wiley & Sons, 1978, pp. 53–65.

8

THE DIAGNOSIS OF MYOCARDIAL INFARCTION

GENERAL CONSIDERATIONS

In retrospect, most patients with acute myocardial infarction have serial changes on their ECGs. Acute changes, however, may be "nonspecific" or not easily recognized. Many factors may interfere with the ability of the ECG to diagnose or localize acute myocardial infarction. As a general rule, a compatible history and *either* diagnostic ECG *or* enzyme changes are required to establish the diagnosis. In the absence of such a history, both diagnostic ECG and enzyme changes should be present in order to establish the diagnosis.

ECG (See Table 8–1, the Localization Chart)

Early Changes—the Hyperacute Tracing

Initial. Peaked T waves in the leads reflecting the involved area (i.e., T vector increased in amplitude and directed toward the infarct).

Subsequent. ST segment elevation ("injury current") in the leads reflecting the involved area (ST vector developing and directed toward the infarct).

Similar changes may be found as a variant of normal ("early repolarization"), or in hyperkalemia.

Usual Transmural Infarction

ST segment elevation > 1 mm initially. Configuration usually straight or convex. Seen in leads reflecting involved area.

T waves. Initially upright and normal; they then flatten and invert in leads reflecting the involved area within hours to days of the acute event.

Q waves. Usually develop over the first 1–2 days after acute transmural infarction. Must be > 0.03 sec in duration. Loss of R waves may be a "Q equivalent" and may depend on the physician's recognition of the range of normal and of the previous R wave amplitude in the affected area.

In true posterior infarction, the inverse of the above change is seen in lead V1, that is, increased amplitude of R wave development.

Table 8–1. LOCALIZATION OF INFARCTION ON ECG

LEADS	LOCATION
2, 3, AVF	inferior
1, AVL	high lateral
V1—V2	anteroseptal
V3, V4	anterior
V5, V6	lateral or apical
V1	posterior

Note: There may be little correspondence between ECG changes and the actual site of necrosis on autopsy, because of cancellation of opposing electrical forces and effects of previous injury.

Localization. May not conform to strict anatomic locations. Q wave alone associated with a high false-positive diagnosis rate, particularly in lead III alone, or III and AVF.

Evolution. Particularly helpful in completing the ECG diagnosis and in recognizing extension of reinfarction. ST segment elevation beyond 3 weeks raises the possibility of a significant ventricular aneurysm. T waves may normalize within the first year. Q waves, on occasion, may disappear in the year following infarction. While generally conceded to represent transmural damage, Q waves may appear transiently during severe ischemia.

Nontransmural Infarction ("Subendocardial")

Traditionally diagnosed when ST depression followed by T inversion occurs, in the absence of the development of Q waves or R wave changes. May also be diagnosed when ST segment elevation and T inversion occur (without QRS changes), or when no diagnostic ECG changes are seen in the presence of a compatible history and diagnostic enzyme elevation.

"Ischemia"

Definition—A reversible state, characterized by transient ECG changes, negative enzymes, and usually a history of brief (< 30 min) chest pain symptoms.

ECG changes. During pain symptoms—ST depression (occasionally elevation). If severe or prolonged, T wave inversion. Following pain relief—prompt resolution (within minutes) of ST segment changes. Return of ST segment to baseline within several hours; T waves may remain inverted for up to 3 days.

Extension/Reinfarction

Definition—Following stabilization or normal evolution of the ECG, any additional elevation of ST segments or inversion of T waves is a *possible* extension or reinfarction. The diagnosis requires secondary enzyme elevations and is usually associated with a compatible history.

Asymptomatic T wave inversions in the area contiguous to the acute MI sometimes occur and are not associated with enzyme

Table 8–2. SERUM ENZYMES IN ACUTE MYOCARDIAL INFARCTION

	TIME FROM ONSET OF SYMPTOMS CAUSED BY ACUTE MYOCARDIAL INFARCTION		
	To Rise Above Normal	**To Peak**	**To Return to Normal**
CK	4–8 hr	12–20 hr	3–4 days
CK-MB	4–8 hr	12–20 hr	2–3 days
SGOT	8–12 hr	18–36 hr	3–4 days
LDH	24–48 hr	3–6 days	8–18 days

changes; they should be considered "contiguous ischemia" rather than extension.

Cardiac Enzymes

General Considerations

To prove useful in the diagnosis of acute myocardial infarction, serum enzymes must rise above the upper limits of normal of the laboratory performing the analysis and must peak and trough in a pattern characteristic of acute myocardial infarction. The time course of enzyme elevation is illustrated in Table 8–2.

Sites of Enzyme Release

Each of the major cardiac enzymes (SGOT, LDH, CK) is also present in other organs and may be released into the circulation as a result of trauma, altered physiology, or a disease state that may simulate the enzymatic appearance of acute myocardial infarction. These medical conditions causing enzyme elevations and their typical patterns are listed in Table 8–3.

Isoenzymes

Definition—Chemically identical enzymes that differ in their movement in an electrophoretic field owing to different stoichiometric configurations.

Lactate dehydrogenase (LDH). Five isoenzymes are recognized. Heart contains primarily LDH_1, while liver and skeletal muscle contain primarily LDH_4 and LDH_5. Red blood cells contain LDH_1, and hemolysis will result in false elevation. Since under normal circumstances $LDH_2 > LDH_1$, reversals of this relationship may be cited as additional evidence of acute myocardial infarction.

HBD (hydroxybutyrate dehydrogenase). Another measure of LDH_1, actually the ability of LDH_1 to reduce alpha-ketobutyric acid. Increases in the serum activity of HBD are seen to parallel LDH_1 activity and may be used in place of the LDH isoenzyme fractionation.

Creatine kinase (CK). Three isoenzymes are identified (MM, MB, BB). Sources are listed in Table 8–3. For all practical

Table 8–3. ENZYME SOURCE AND NONCORONARY CAUSES OF ENZYME ELEVATION

	SOURCES OF ENZYME	MEDICAL CONDITIONS ASSOCIATED WITH RISE OF ENZYME
CK	Heart, skeletal muscle, (brain and GI tract in very small quantities)	Myocarditis, pericarditis, cardiac trauma, muscular dystrophy, muscle trauma, alcohol intoxication, diabetes mellitus (with or without ketosis), convulsions, psychosis, intramuscular injections
CK-MB	Heart	Muscular dystrophy, myocarditis, pericarditis
SGOT	Liver, heart, skeletal muscle, lung	CHF, tachyarrhythmias with rates > 140 for > 30 minutes, DC countershock, myocarditis, IM injections, use of oral contraceptives, pulmonary embolism, shock, liver disease, pericarditis
LDH	Liver, heart, skeletal muscle, kidney, red and white blood cells	Hemolysis, megaloblastic anemia, leukemia, chronic liver disease, renal infarction, pulmonary embolism, shock, severe exercise

purposes, elevation of serum MB may be considered indicative of myocardial cellular injury.

Practical considerations include (1) MB generally falls faster than total CK and is usually within normal range by 48–72 hours after infarction, at a time when total CK *is still elevated.* Thus, an isoenzyme determination performed near or after this time may show *elevation* of total CK without MB elevation. (2) MB isoenzyme is heat labile and must be either promptly analyzed by the laboratory or kept cooled within 2 hours after drawing. Deterioration of the sample will occur at room temperature and is another reason for false-negative MB determination.

Serum Myoglobin

Myoglobin lost from injured myocardial cells appears in both serum and urine following myocardial infarction. Myoglobin appears earlier than CK (as early as 3 hours after onset of symptoms). While theoretically attractive for detection of myocardial damage shortly after acute myocardial infarction, its appearance in the serum in brief bursts and its release from skeletal muscle limit its clinical usefulness.

Other Laboratory Measures

Sedimentation Rate. Rises within a few days. Remains elevated for several weeks. Of little clinical usefulness.

White Blood Cell Count. Rises within a few hours, generally to levels of 12,000–15,000 and occasionally to 20,000. A "shift to the left" in polymorphonuclear leukocytes usually accompanies the rise.

Hemoglobin/Hematocrit Levels. Usually rise during the first few days, as a result of hemoconcentration.

Chest Radiograph

General Considerations. Should be taken early after admission to evaluate heart size and pulmonary vasculature as an index of cardiac compensation. There is a direct correlation between increasing abnormalities of heart size and pulmonary congestive changes on this initial evaluation and survival at 1 month and 1 year (Battler et al.).

Technique. In most institutions, patients with suspected acute coronary symptoms have a chest radiograph taken by portable technique, frequently with the patient in a supine position. Evaluation of heart size and pulmonary vasculature is usually difficult or impossible on such films. A 6 foot PA portable film of better quality and usually comparable to a standard film can be obtained as follows: (1) have patient sit upright at edge of bed; (2) film cassette is held in front of chest by patient, with lower edge resting on legs; (3) portable x-ray machine is located 6 feet behind patient, and film is obtained PA. Care must be taken to assure that x-ray beam is perpendicular to patient and that beam is aimed away from personnel or other patients (for example, directed at the outer wall of patient's room).

X-ray–Cardiac Status Discrepancies (Kostuk Effect). A diagnostic lag (acute cardiac decompensation lagging behind radiographic changes) of up to 12 hours may occur. A therapeutic lag (resolution of decompensation lagging behind x-ray resolution) of 1–4 days may also occur.

REFERENCES

Battler A, Karlinger JS, Higgins CB, et al: The initial chest x-ray in acute myocardial infarction: Prediction of early and late mortality and survival. Circulation *61*:1004, 1980.

Roberts R, Gowda KS, Ludbrook PA, Sobel BE: The specificity of elevated serum MJV CPK activity in the diagnosis of acute myocardial infarction. Am J Cardiol *36*:433, 1975.

Sobel BE, Shell WE: Serum enzyme determinations in the diagnosis and assessment of myocardial infarction. Circulation *45*:471, 1972.

Varki AP, Roby DS, Watts H, Zatuchni J: Serum myoglobin in acute myocardial infarction: A clinical study and review of the literature. Am Heart J *96*:680, 1978.

9

THE DIAGNOSIS OF UNSTABLE ANGINA

Features on the History

Definition. Unstable angina is either new in onset or superimposed on chronic stable angina and is characterized by its (1) increasing severity, frequency, or duration and/or decreasing responsiveness to nitroglycerin, or (2) by its occurrence at rest or with minimal exertion.

New-onset angina that does not fulfill the above criteria is best excluded from this categorization.

Character. Similar to typical stable angina, although usually more severe or widely radiating and more likely to have associated diaphoresis, nausea, and apprehension.

Duration of Pain. Usually less than 30 minutes. Continuing pain of more than 45 minutes is more typically associated with acute MI and should be treated as such.

Synonyms. Also called preinfarction angina, crescendo angina, intermediate coronary syndrome. While at greater risk of acute myocardial infarction, most patients with unstable angina do not progress to it and the term *unstable* is best used.

Physical Findings

Of little help in establishing the diagnosis. If the significance of observed chest discomfort is uncertain, an ischemic etiology may be inferred by the transient appearance (during an episode) of a paradoxically split S2, S3 or S4 gallop, the murmur of mitral regurgitation (MR), or a dyskinetic apical impulse.

Laboratory Findings

ECG Changes

ST segment deviations, either depression or elevation, occur during discomfort and partly or totally remit with relief.

T wave inversion during episodes of chest discomfort may occur.

Occasionally, ST and T wave abnormalities may be absent. The diagnosis must then be inferred on the basis of the history. The presence of known coronary artery disease (CAD) further reinforces the clinical diagnosis. Therapy should usually await the development of ECG changes (see Chapter 8).

Exercise stress testing, because of the possibility of inducing acute myocardial infarction, is contraindicated until medical stability is achieved or coronary artery disease excluded by coronary arteriography.

Serum Cardiac Enzymes

Levels should remain within the normal range, although they may rise and fall within the normal range. However, recent reports now indicate that minimal elevation (CK and/or CK-MB) above normal represents small (or "patchy") infarction, although release of enzyme by ischemic cells also may occur.

Other

Other laboratory findings of myocardial cell necrosis (increased WBC count, increased ESR) are absent.

Etiology

Transient increase in O_2 demand—increased blood pressure may precede pain and ST changes.

Transient decrease of O_2 supply—coronary spasm. Definite and unprovoked coronary spasm occurs, and may result in angina at rest. Spasm also has been shown to occur in the setting of acute MI (Maseri et al). Patients with spasm may have ST segment depression or elevation and may have normal coronary arteries or fixed (atherosclerotic) coronary artery lesions. Exercise, handgrip, or cold may provoke spasm.

There is insufficient evidence to establish which of these two mechanisms is primary in unstable angina, or whether the two mechanisms may work in concert.

Physical or emotional factors may provoke a change in the character of angina and may be responsible for a patient presenting symptoms resembling the unstable angina syndrome.

Coronary Artery Lesions

Increased incidence of main left coronary artery stenosis (Alison et al): 13%. This is in contrast to pathologic studies that confirm an overall incidence of 7% in unselected coronary patients.

Distribution of coronary lesions otherwise similar to that in patients with chronic stable angina.

Prognosis

What proportion of patients with unstable angina has new-onset angina, a crescendo pattern superimposed on chronic, stable angina, or rest angina depends on the series of patients studied as well as how investigators defined the syndrome at the time of study. The prospective study performed by Gazes et al is most instructive, since it provides a baseline for the natural history of the disease before surgical intervention was commonplace. These investigators followed 140 patients over a 10 year period and found a 5 year survival rate of 61% and a cumulative 10 year survival rate of 48%. Most patients of Gazes and associates were not treated with beta-blocking agents, since these drugs were not available until the end of the study. All their patients were treated with a combination of rest, nitrates, sedatives, and diet, and a majority were treated with anticoagulants (either warfarin or heparin).Twenty-one per cent of their patients developed acute myocardial infarction within 8 months of the onset of their unstable angina syndrome, and, of these patients, 41% had fatal infarctions. A high-risk subgroup, defined as having persistent pain in the hospital and documented ischemic ST changes during pain with a history of prior stable angina, revealed a 1 year survival rate of 57% and a 5 year survival rate of 27%. Thirty-five per cent of this subgroup developed a myocardial infarction within 3 months of the onset of the accelerated phase of their illness, with a mortality rate of 63% during that subsequent myocardial infarction.

This study identifies several critical factors upon which today's therapy of unstable angina should be based (see Chapter 17). First, acceleration of angina is a critical variable in the natural history of coronary artery disease and carries with it a risk markedly greater than that of chronic stable angina.

Patients appear to present the greatest risk if they continue to have angina after admission to the hospital, despite routine administration of opiate analgesics, sedation, use of nitrates, and control of hypertension.

Second, while an increased risk continues for at least 10 years after the onset of symptoms of unstable angina, the *highest* risk for recurrent MI or death occurs during the first 2 years. This trend suggests that there was some natural selection of the remaining patients, who exhibited a relatively good prognosis in later years.

Other important areas of controversy include the pathophysiology of rest angina, particularly the difference between episodes associated with ST segment elevation and those associated with ST segment depression. There remains a difference of opinion regarding the prognosis between medically treated patients and surgically treated patients. Studies comparing the coronary anatomic patterns of patients with unstable angina and those of patients with stable angina have revealed no significant differences, except for, perhaps, a dearth of collateral vessels in patients with unstable angina and a larger percentage of patients with left mainstem coronary artery lesions.

Several reports have addressed the clinical and angiographic significance of the direction of the ST segment shift on the resting ECG in patients with unstable angina. These studies, including a large prospective National Heart, Lung, and Blood Institute randomized trial of unstable angina, failed to discern any appreciable differences in myocardial infarction rate and in-hospital mortality between patients who underwent medical versus urgent surgical therapy. In fact, it was concluded that the subgroup of patients with ST segment elevation behaved no differently from the larger subgroup of patients with ST segment depression with respect to in-hospital myocardial infarction and mortality. Thus, the weight of evidence to date appears not to support the thesis that surgery influences the early hospital course of patients with unstable angina more favorably than does intensive medical therapy.

Of course, an exceedingly high percentage of patients in both the nonrandomized and randomized trials of unstable angina have "crossed over" to surgical therapy for the relief of unremitting angina, and there is little question that surgical therapy is more likely to improve the symptoms of accelerating angina. Thus, it is difficult to obtain comparable long-term follow-up data on many patients who have had medical and surgical therapy because of the significantly high surgical cross-over rate. It would be hard to predict what would have been the outcome had medical therapy been pursued further.

Prinzmetal Variant Angina

Definition: anginal pain at rest, associated with episodic ST segment elevation.

Extent of coronary disease and prognosis do not differ from the group of unstable angina patients as a whole.

Now considered to be a manifestation of coronary artery spasm with or without superimposed atherosclerotic CAD.

REFERENCES

Alison HW, Russel RO, Mantel JA, et al: Coronary anatomy and arteriography in patients with unstable angina pectoris. Am J Cardiol *41*:204, 1978.

Braunwald E: Coronary spasm and an acute myocardial infarction—new possibility for treatment and prevention (Editorial). N Engl J Med *299*:1301, 1978.

Buston A, Goldberg S, Harken A, et al: Coronary artery spasm immediately after myocardial revascularization: Recognition and treatment. N Engl J Med *304*:1249, 1981.

Gazes PC, Mobley EM, Faris H, et al: Preinfarction (unstable) angina—a prospective study. Ten year follow up. Circulation *48*:331, 1973.

Maseri A, Severi S, DeNes M, et al: "Variant angina": One aspect of a continuous spectrum of vasospastic myocardial ischemia. Am J Cardiol *42*:1019, 1978.

Prinzmetal M, Kennamer R, Merliss R, et al: Angina pectoris I. A variant form of angina pectoris. Am J Med *27*:375, 1959.

Scheidt S, Wolk M, Killip T: Unstable angina pectoris: Natural history, hemodynamics, uncertainties of treatment and the ethics of clinical study. Am J Med *60*:409, 1976.

Unstable Angina Pectoris; national study group to compare medical and surgical therapy. I. Am J Cardiol *37*:896, 1976; II. Am J Cardiol *42*:839, 1978; III. Am J Cardiol *45*:819, 1980.

10

ECHOCARDIOGRAPHY AND RADIONUCLIDE IMAGING IN MYOCARDIAL INFARCTION DIAGNOSIS

ECHOCARDIOGRAPHY

General Considerations

Although echocardiography is an extremely valuable technique for evaluating cardiac chamber size and wall thickness, valvular disease, and overall ventricular function, its ability in assessing quantitative regional left ventricular wall motion in acute myocardial ischemia and infarction is limited, because M-mode echocardiography images small segments of the interventricular septum and posterior left ventricular free wall (Fig. 10–1). Thus, regional wall motion abnormalities and even left ventricular aneurysms—particularly those involving the anterior wall of the left ventricle—may be missed completely.

Since ischemia may induce distortions of left ventricular geometry by chamber dilatation or regional dyssynergy, ultrasonically obtained global ventricular function may be inaccurate and misleading. Thus, limitations inherent in the ability of M-mode ultrasound to evaluate the entire chamber silhouette may result in inappropriate assumptions about the presence or absence of segmental dyssynergy, as well as potential over- and underestimations of left ventricular ejection fraction. These criticisms, in general, are less applicable to two-dimensional echocardiography, which provides 30 to 90 degree sector format tomographic images of several planes of left ventricular myocardium (Fig. 10–2).

Clinical Applications

Despite these methodologic difficulties, important information about left ventricular function can be obtained in patients with acute or old myocardial infarction. Abnormalities of left ventricular contraction corresponding to the site of infarction localized by electrocardiogram have been shown to occur in 84% of cases in one series. In addition, an increased left ventricular internal dimension was observed in 50% of acute infarct patients, which correlated closely with clinical, hemodynamic, and angiographic signs of heart failure.

Echocardiography has been extremely useful in delineating small pericardial effusions in patients with late, autoimmune postinfarc-

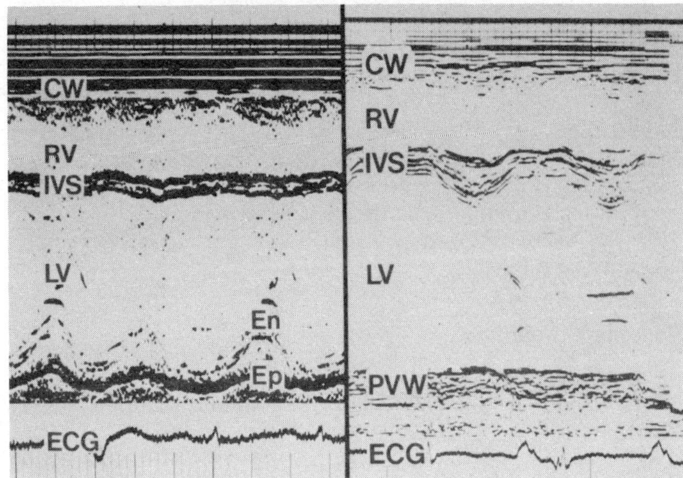

Figure 10–1. M-mode recordings of anterior (left) and posterior (right) myocardial infarctions. In both cases, the affected myocardium is akinetic and the contralateral wall moves vigorously. CW, chest wall; ECG, electrocardiogram; En, endocardium; Ep, epicardium; IVS, interventricular septum; LV, left ventricle; PVW, posterior ventricular wall; RV, right ventricle. (From Leech G, Kisslo J: Geigy Series on Echocardiography (2nd Series); Unit 3, Heart Muscle Disease. Summit, NJ, Geigy Phamaceuticals, 1982.)

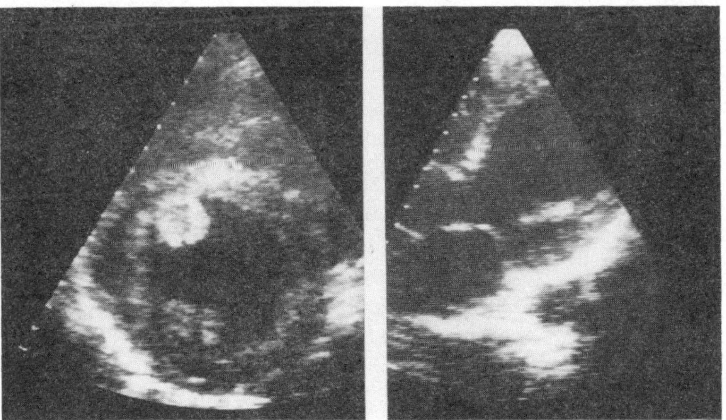

Figure 10–2. *Left:* 2-D parasternal long axis view in systole following myocardial infarction. *Right:* 2-D parasternal short axis view of left ventricle following transmural myocardial infarction. A mural thrombus (white echodense mass) is present. (From Leech G, Kisslo J: Geigy Series on Echocardiography (2nd Series); Unit 3, Heart Muscle Disease. Summit, NJ, Geigy Pharmaceuticals, 1982.)

tion pericarditis (Dressler's syndrome), which is discussed in Chapter 22.

Other uses for echocardiography in the setting of acute ischemic heart disease include

a) the noninvasive diagnosis of right ventricular infarction (discussed in Chapter 20), in which M-mode echocardiography characteristically shows increased right ventricular end-diastolic chamber dimension (i.e., dilatation) and an increased ratio of right-to-left ventricular end-diastolic chamber dimension; and

b) demonstration of interventricular septum rupture postinfarction in some patients (see Chapter 21).

Recommendations

Partially useful in assessing septal and posterior wall infarction.

Less helpful in assessing anterior wall motion abnormalities, or aneurysm.

M-mode echocardiography may provide qualitative information about regional and global left ventricular function following infarction, but a quantified assessment of regional and overall ejection fraction can be obtained with radionuclide imaging techniques (discussion to follow).

Useful for detecting pericardial effusion post-MI and, in some cases, rupture of the interventricular septum or right ventricular infarction.

RADIONUCLIDE IMAGING

Myocardial Scintigraphy with Infarct-Avid Radiopharmaceuticals

General Considerations

During the last decade, positive "hot-spot" myocardial scintigraphic methods have become available for the non-invasive assessment of myocardial infarction, utilizing a variety of different radiopharmaceuticals, including technetium–99m–tetracycline (Tc–99m–SN), technetium–99m–glucoheptonate, gallium–67 citrate, and, most notably, technetium–99m–stannous pyrophosphate (Tc–99m–PYP). With hot-spot myocardial imaging, the abnormal area is visualized as a region of avid *increased* radioactivity (Fig. 10–3). These scintigraphic agents can be used not only to detect presence, location, and size of infarction but also to determine whether a myocardial infarction is acute or old.

Tc–99m–PYP embodies the ideal physical characteristics of a radioisotope (Tc–99m) combined with a phosphate complex (PYP) that is rapidly cleared from the blood, allowing myocardial imaging as early as 1 hour after injection. There is avid accumulation of the radionuclide in the region of acutely infarcted myocardium,

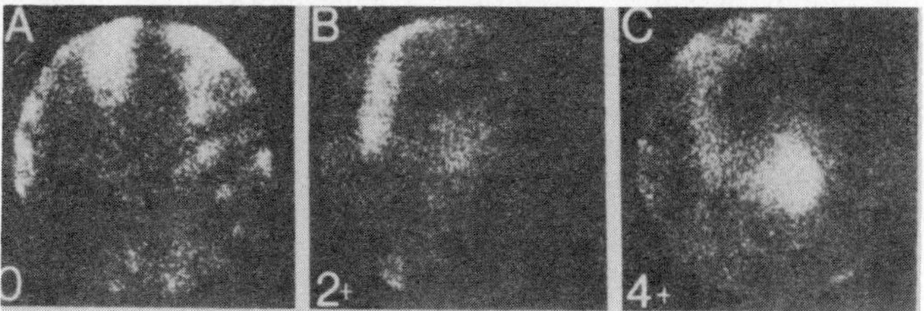

Figure 10–3. Typical images obtained from technetium pyrophosphate scintigrams in a normal (grade 0) patient without acute infarction (Panel *A*) and in patients with MI (Panels *B* and *C*). A 2^+ myocardial scintigram (Panel B) represents an abnormal, diffuse uptake of radiopharmaceutical with the faintest but definitely increased uptake of technetium that one can detect. A 4^+ scan (Panel C) indicates focal myocardial uptake greater than adjacent bone activity. Technetium scans graded 2^+ to 4^+ are considered positive for myocardial necrosis (see text).

with high activity ratios between infarcted and adjacent normal myocardium. Despite the fact that Tc–99m–PYP accumulates in bone, there is no significant liver accumulation, and, as a result, inferior wall myocardial infarction can be visualized without difficulty.

Positive Tc–99m–PYP scintigrams relate to the incorporation of the pyrophosphate moiety into the hydroxyapatite crystalline structure present within damaged myocardial cells. Most investigators believe that a portion of the damaged cells must be irreversibly injured, or necrotic, before they will concentrate pyrophosphate. However, there is as yet no universal agreement on the significance of diffuse and faintly positive radionuclide uptake, since these "equivocal" patterns have been observed in nontransmural infarction, in unstable angina, and in chronically ischemic myocardium. There are probably three types of abnormal study (Table 10–1):

(1) Acute transmural infarction with a focal increase (3+ to 4+) in radioactivity in necrotic myocardium (Fig. 10–3);

(2) Acute, nontransmural infarction with a focal or diffuse increase (2+) in radioactivity in ischemic left ventricular myocardium;

Table 10–1. CRITERIA FOR Tc-99m-PYP SCINTIGRAPHIC ASSESSMENT OF ACUTE MYOCARDIAL INFARCTION

DEGREE OF UPTAKE IN THE REGION OF THE MYOCARDIUM	
4+	Greatest intensity
3+	Equal to bone intensity
2+	Moderate
1+	Slight
0	Nonvisualized
INTERPRETATION ON THE BASIS OF MYOCARDIAL UPTAKE	
0 to 1+	Negative
3 to 4+	Positive
2+ Focal	Positive
2+ Diffuse	Equivocal

(3) Equivocal studies, comprising individuals with apparent blood pool radioactivity (2+•diffuse uptake) that is intermediate between patients described in No. 2 and normal. Probably most "false-positive" studies occur in this group; indeed, in one study of 235 patients with acute chest pain syndromes, 35 of 50 patients (70%) with such equivocal scans had no evidence of acute myocardial infarction.

Clinical Applications

The time course of abnormal Tc–99m–PYP uptake after acute myocardial infarction is predicated on acute myocardial necrosis and some residual blood flow to the infarcted area; this permits differentiation between acute infarction and remote infarction. Infarct-avid Tc–99m–PYP scintigrams become positive at 12–36 hours, with the degree of increased uptake reaching a maximum between 48–72 hours after the acute event. Thereafter, the degree of uptake lessens, although the scan may remain positive for 5–6 days. Usually, 1 week after infarction the Tc–99m–PYP scan is negative, although recent data suggest that in as many as 40–50% of cases, some residual uptake persists for an indefinite time period after acute infarction. Some evidence suggests that patients who exhibit such "residual scan positivity" may have a more unfavorable long-term prognosis following acute infarction.

From a practical standpoint, however, Tc–99m–PYP scans have not been as helpful in diagnosing acute infarction as initially expected. For example, in acute transmural infarction (which is readily diagnosed by electrocardiographic Q waves and positive cardiac enzymes), a markedly positive scan with a 3+ to 4+ focal uptake adds little to the diagnosis. In contrast, the more subtle nontransmural infarction (often associated with equivocal ECG and cardiac enzyme changes) is frequently difficult to detect with the Tc–99m–PYP technique, may exhibit faint (2+) focal or diffuse uptake, and may not distinguish acute subendocardial necrosis.

It appears that the greatest clinical utility for Tc–99m–PYP scans in the setting of acute myocardial ischemia is when the ECG and/or the cardiac enzymes are obscured. Examples are the patient with acute chest pain and left bundle branch block on ECG, or the patient whose chest pain occurred more than 24–48 hours prior to admission, in whom the time course of biochemical necrosis (i.e., cardiac enzyme pattern) may have elapsed.

Finally, it is important to mention the clinical conditions that have, on occasion, been associated with "false-positive" Tc–99m–PYP scans: (1) unstable angina pectoris, (2) calcified cardiac valves, (3) left ventricular aneurysm, (4) old myocardial infarction, (5) postelectrical cardioversion, and (6) healing rib fractures.

Recommendations

For acute, infarct-avid myocardial scintigraphy:

(1) To assess acute infarction in the presence of left bundle branch block or in other conditions in which ECG abnormalities may obscure or preclude the diagnosis of acute infarction;

(2) To assess acute infarction when the time course of cardiac enzymes or isoenzymes is unclear; e.g., enzymes that have returned to baseline;

(3) To distinguish a nontransmural infarction from unstable angina (rarely diagnostic).

Cold-Spot Myocardial Perfusion Imaging

General Considerations

Myocardial perfusion scintigraphy with radiopharmaceuticals (potassium–43, rubidium–81, and thallium–201) is characterized by *decreased* uptake in abnormal myocardial regions, so-called "cold spot" imaging. Although cold-spot scintigraphic studies have been employed in patients with acute coronary artery disease, the most widespread application of this imaging technique has been in the population with chronic ischemic heart disease. The utility of thallium–201 myocardial perfusion imaging in distinguishing ischemia from infarction during exercise and redistribution will not be discussed here.

Cold-spot scintigraphy has diagnostic usefulness in acute myocardial infarction. If obtained early after the acute event, this technique has high sensitivity for acute infarction. If several days elapse between an infarction and thallium–201 imaging, the sensitivity decreases, especially in the case of inferior wall myocardial infarctions. Therefore, a completely normal cold-spot scintigram (entirely homogeneous tracer uptake) within the initial 24 hours of suspected infarction may provide clinically useful and relevant data (Fig. 10–4). However, thallium–201 scintigraphy cannot differentiate old and acute infarctions. Thus, the presence of an abnormality in the setting of suspected acute infarction does not necessarily confirm the diagnosis.

Clinical Application (See also Chapter 17)

As discussed, the major purpose of thallium-201 scintigraphy applies to its concomitant use with exercise testing, especially in patients in whom the more traditional noninvasive studies are inconclusive. Such clinical conditions include

chest pain with abnormal resting ECG;

chest pain with normal coronary arteriography;

coronary disease screening in asymptomatic patients with abnormal stress electrocardiograms;

evaluation of the functional significance and extent of coronary artery disease;

evaluation of chest pain following aortocoronary bypass surgery; and

assessment of acute myocardial infarction.

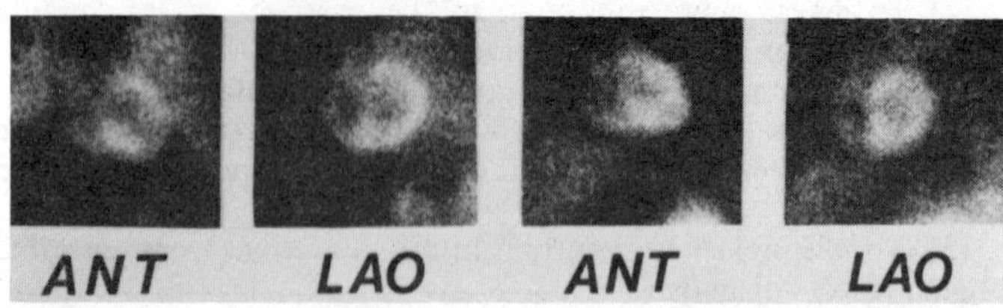

Figure 10–4. The far left thallium scintigram obtained in the anterior (ANT) projection reveals an extensive perfusion defect (decreased uptake or "cold spot") of the anterior wall of the left ventricle; in the left anterior oblique (LAO) projection (second left), evidence for decreased perfusion of the interventricular septum is seen. These findings are consistent with an acute anteroseptal MI and can be compared with the corresponding normal thallium perfusion scintigrams in the ANT (second right) and LAO (far right) views.

Since the purpose of this chapter is to discuss the role of thallium–201 imaging in the CCU, we will address only the first and last conditions.

In patients with an abnormal resting ECG (left bundle branch block [LBBB], left ventricular hypertrophy [LVH], digitalis administration, etc.), the diagnosis of acute myocardial infarction may be difficult. In such individuals, cold-spot scintigraphy may demonstrate an area of reduced myocardial perfusion that could facilitate the diagnosis of infarction.

As discussed, resting thallium–201 scintigrams obtained later than 1 day after suspected infarction—especially nontransmural infarction—are not likely to detect the presence of acute myocardial infarction.

Recommendations

For diagnosis of acute myocardial infarction:

(1) Resting thallium–201 scintigraphy may be useful in patients with an abnormal resting ECG, in whom the abnormality (LBBB, LVH, digitalis effect) may obscure the diagnosis of acute infarction.

(2) When thallium–201 imaging is performed within 24 hours of suspected acute infarction, the technique has a high sensitivity for acute infarction. However, small, nontransmural infarctions may escape detection, and this method cannot distinguish acute from old infarction. A completely normal scan makes the diagnosis of infarction unlikely.

Radionuclide Angiography

General Considerations

In the preceding sections, we described radionuclide methods for imaging the myocardium and their application to the diagnosis of acute myocardial ischemia and infarction. Radionuclide angiography, in contrast, provides quantification of ventricular function and segmental wall motion by imaging the cardiac blood pool. With these techniques, global and regional ventricular performance, cardiac chamber anatomy, and intracardiac shunts can be derived.

Two techniques are currently available for clinical use: the first-pass cardiac blood pool scintigram and the gated equilibrium blood pool scan. Detailed description of these two techniques is beyond the scope of this manual. However, both techniques provide accurate, noninvasive measurement of global and regional ejection fraction, and, as a result, segmental and overall left *and* right ventricular wall motion can be assessed with the type of precision that rivals invasive left ventricular angiography. Figure 10–5 is an example of the normal left and right ejection fraction images obtained during gated equilibrium blood pool imaging.

Both the gated equilibrium radionuclide angiogram and the first-pass cardiac blood pool scan afford accurate measurement of global ejection fraction, and correlation between the two methods, as well as with standard cineangiography, is high (r = 0.87–0.89). Other hemodynamic indices (such as peak ejection rate) require high temporal resolution of the left ventricular time activity curve, which cannot be adequately assessed by first-pass studies. Similarly, regional wall motion can be quantified with either method, but the high counting rate achieved with gated equilibrium scintigraphy provides improved accuracy and optimal spatial resolution, particularly when regional ejection fraction is measured.

Equilibrium studies are superior to the first-pass technique for patient monitoring and the performance of sequential studies. Studies can be performed for up to 4 hours after injection of the radiopharmaceutical, permitting imaging in multiple views and after either physiologic or pharmacologic interventions. Equilibrium studies require 2 to 3 minutes (approximately 300,000 counts) for adequate imaging, which may be difficult with an unstable or agitated patient. In contrast, first-pass studies require separate radiopharmaceutical injections each time imaging is performed, require only 5 or 6 cardiac cycles, and may be preferable for acute studies in unstable patients or when rapid changes in cardiac physiology are anticipated with interventions.

Clinical Applications

Radionuclide angiography is an extremely useful, noninvasive method for quantifying cardiac hemodynamics and global/regional wall motion and ejection fraction. A variety of applications in the assessment of acute coronary disease have been developed.

Acute Myocardial Infarction. Early after infarction, radionuclide angiography can be used to assess the extent of abnormal, global left ventricular pump performance, as well as the extent of abnormal segmental wall motion, providing important prognostic information (Figs. 10–6 and 10–7).

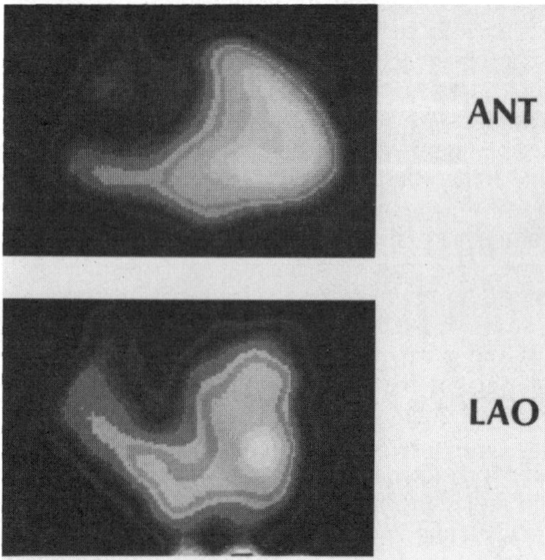

Figure 10–5. These functional normal ejection fraction images of a gated cardiac blood pool scan, obtained in the anterior (ANT) and left anterior oblique (LAO) projections, illustrate the normal, intact wall motion seen in a patient without global or regional left ventricular dysfunction. The "gray scale" of the picture elements (pixels) depicted here correlates with the degree of maintained or disturbed heart function (white/light gray = normal; dary gray = hypokinetic/akinetic).

In addition, radionuclide angiography can be used to assess the presence of concomitant right ventricular infarction—especially in the setting of inferior wall infarction. Finally, these techniques permit assessment of ventricular chamber dimension and indirect measurement of cardiac output.

Congestive Heart Failure and Chronic Coronary Artery Disease. Radionuclide angiography can be used to differentiate patients with segmental left ventricular dysfunction (localized akinesis or dyskinesis) from patients with diffuse left ventricular hypokinesis, but this application will not be discussed in detail here.

Other clinical applications, beyond the scope of discussion here, include

the effect of exercise on global and regional ventricular performance in patients with ischemic heart disease;

the effects of drug interventions on ventricular performance;

the definition of cardiovascular pathoanatomy (pericardial effusion, idiopathic hypertrophic subaortic stenosis [IHSS], cardiac tumors, etc.); and

intracardiac shunt detection.

Recommendations

It is difficult to provide strict recommendations or guidelines for the use of radionuclide angiography in patients with acute ischemic

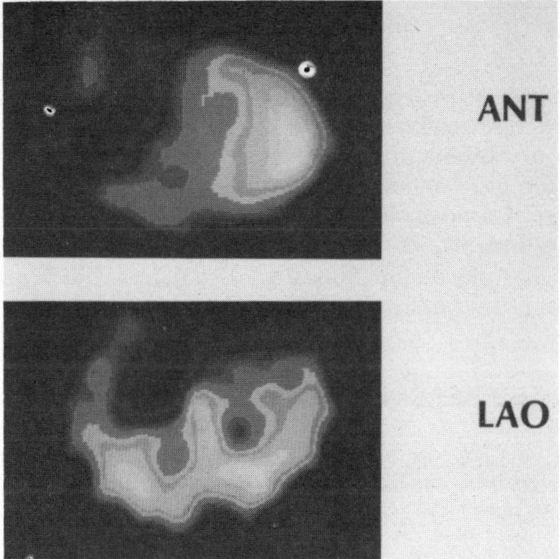

Figure 10–6. These functional images were obtained in a patient with a recent transmural, inferior wall MI. Regional wall motion is entirely normal in the LAO projection (normal "gray scale") but in the ANT view is abnormal (dark gray = hypokinetic/akinetic) in the basal portion of the inferior wall.

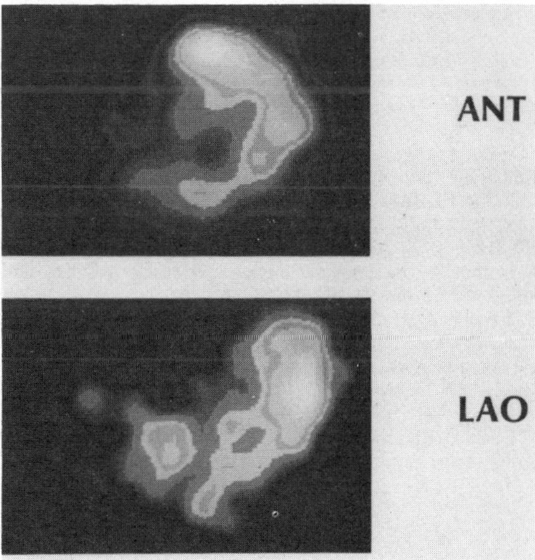

Figure 10–7. These functional images were obtained in a patient with an inferior wall MI and more extensive segmental wall motion abnormalities than in the patient shown in Figure 10–6. In the ANT view, the basal portion of the inferior wall is frankly akinetic (dark gray), while the distal inferior wall is hypokinetic. In the LAO view, significant akinesis of the basal (upper) septal region and, to a lesser degree, the distal (lower) septum is seen. These regional wall motion abnormalities are consistent with an inferoseptal infarction.

heart disease at this time. Both first-pass and gated equilibrium techniques have advantages and limitations, but both provide accurate assessment of global and regional ejection fraction in patients too ill to undergo invasive catheterization.

The use of a portable scintillation camera and gating device, in combination with a computer, will facilitate the bedside quantification of ventricular function in CCU patients with acute myocardial ischemia and infarction.

SUGGESTED READING

Berman DS, Amsterdam EA, Hines HH: New approach to interpretation of Technetium–99m pyrophosphate scintigraphy in detection of acute myocardial infarction. Am J Cardiol *39*:341, 1977.

Bodenheimer M, Banka VS, Helfont R: Nuclear cardiology. I. Radionuclide angiographic assessment of left ventricular contraction: Uses, limitations and future directions. Am J Cardiol *45*:73, 1980.

Corya BC, Rasmussen S, Knoebel SB, et al: Echocardiography in acute myocardial infarction. Am J Cardiol *36*:1, 1975.

Feigenbaum H, Corya BC, Dillon JC, et al: Role of echocardiography in patients with coronary artery disease. Am J Cardiol *37*:775, 1976.

Holman BL: Radioisotopic examination of the cardiovascular system, *In* Braunwald E (ed.): Heart Disease: A Textbook of Cardiovascular Medicine. Philadelphia, W. B. Saunders Company, 1980.

Maddox DE, Holman DE, Wynne J, et al: Ejection fraction image: A non-invasive index of regional left ventricular wall motion. Am J Cardiol *41*:1230, 1978.

Maddox DE, Wynne J, Uren R, et al: Regional ejection fraction: A quantitative radionuclide index of regional left ventricular performance. Circulation *59*:1001, 1979.

Mason DT, DeMaria AN, Berman DS: Principles of Non-Invasive Cardiac Imaging: Echocardiography and Nuclear Cardiology. New York, LeJacq Publishing, 1980.

Parkey RW, Bonte FJ, Buja LM, Willerson JT (eds): Clinical Nuclear Cardiology. New York, Appleton-Century-Crofts, 1979.

Schelbert HR, Henning H, Asburn WL, et al: Serial measurements of left ventricular ejection fraction by radionuclide angiography early and late after myocardial infarction. Am J Cardiol *38*:407, 1976.

Teicholz LE, Kreulen T, Herman MV, et al: Problems in echocardiographic volume determinations; echocardiographic-angiographic correlations in the absence of asynergy. Am J Cardiol *37*:7, 1976.

Wackers FJT, Lie KI, Liem KL, et al: Thallium–201 scintigraphy in unstable angina pectoris. Circulation *57*:738, 1978.

Wackers FJT, Sokole EB, Samson G, et al: Value and limitations of Thallium–201 scintigraphy in the acute phase of myocardial infarction. N Engl J Med *295*:1, 1976.

11
PROGNOSIS IN MYOCARDIAL INFARCTION

GENERAL GUIDELINES

Effect on Left Ventricular Dysfunction

It has now been well established that power failure, in the absence of complicating lesions such as mitral regurgitation or ventricular septal defects, occurs strictly in proportion to the quantity of myocardium that is damaged—i.e., in proportion to infarct size. In both experimental and clinical studies, it has been shown that evidence of left ventricular failure exists when approximately 20 to 25% of the left ventricular myocardium is damaged, and that lesions involving more than 40–45% of the left ventricular myocardium are associated with cardiogenic shock and a fatal outcome. Within this range of left ventricular damage—between 25 and 50%—the entire spectrum of heart failure, from mild to severe, becomes clinically apparent.

Several classifications exist for determining prognosis in acute myocardial infarction. Most of these are based on the clinical assessment of left ventricular failure. One of the first attempts at such a clinical classification was formulated by Killip and Kimball in 1967 (Table 11–1). It became apparent, indeed, that hospital mortality was directly related to the severity of left ventricular dysfunction, based on clinical presentation at admission to the CCU. Peel and Norris have developed prognostic indices for patients with acute infarction, based on composite scores derived from a number of different variables (age, sex, past medical history, left ventricular failure, shock, ECG, arrhythmias, heart size). Despite this exacting approach, left ventricular failure heavily weights these two indices in the direction of poor prognosis.

More recently, prognostic indices employing invasive hemodynamic measurements have been utilized. These data have been derived from pulmonary artery (Swan-Ganz) catheterization; they have been employed alone and as part of a multivariate analysis approach. One such prognostic index was derived from the following parameters:

$$\text{Prognostic index} = \frac{\text{DP} \times \text{MVO}_2\ \text{sat}}{\text{PCW}}$$

where DP = cuff diastolic blood pressure; MVO_2 sat = pulmonary arterial blood oxygen saturation; and PCW = pulmonary capillary

Table 11–1. KILLIP CLASSIFICATION IN ACUTE MYOCARDIAL INFARCTION

	DEFINITION OF CLINICAL CLASS	PROPORTION OF PATIENTS ADMITTED TO CCU(%)	HOSPITAL MORTALITY (APPROXIMATE %)
Class I	Absence of rales; no S3 gallop	30–40	6–8
Class II	Rales ≤ 50% of the lung fields *or* and S3 gallop	30–50	25–30
Class III	Rales > 50% of the lung fields; frequently, pulmonary edema	5–10	40–44
Class IV	Cardiogenic shock	10	80–90

(From Killip T III, Kimball JT: Am J Cardiol *20*:459, 1967.)

wedge pressure. The lower the index, the higher the mortality. Patients with an index of ≥ 250 had a 2% mortality, while those with an index of < 250 had a 61% mortality.

The symptoms and signs of heart failure may be subtle and qualitative and, at times, may be difficult to assess accurately at the bedside (Table 11–2). Forrester and coworkers have developed a semiquantitative classification for patients with myocardial infarction based on cardiac output and wedge pressure determinations. They have identified four clinical/hemodynamic subsets (Table 11–3). Subset I patients with normal peripheral perfusion in the absence of pulmonary congestion (normal cardiac output and wedge pressure) had the best prognosis (2.2% mortality), while subset IV patients with both pulmonary congestion and peripheral hypoperfusion (depressed cardiac output below 1.8 L/min/M^2 and wedge pressure greater than 27 mm Hg) had the worst prognosis (56% mortality). Patients with isolated pulmonary congestion (subset II) and isolated peripheral hypoperfusion (subset III) had intermediate prognoses of 10% and 22%, respectively. However, approximately 25% of patients with cardiac indices less than 2.2 L/min/M^2 and 15% of patients with wedge pressures greater than 18 mm Hg are not discernible clinically. Thus, invasive hemodynamic monitoring may be necessary to confirm the appropriate clinical/hemodynamic subset and to initiate appropriate management.

Table 11–2. CLINICAL FEATURES OF LEFT VENTRICULAR FAILURE

BASIS	INCREASED PULMONARY-CAPILLARY PRESSURE	DECREASED CARDIAC INDEX
Subjective	Dyspnea	Obtundation, fatigue
Objective	Rales, x-ray evidence of congestion	Reduced blood pressure, increased heart rate, cold skin and oliguria

Table 11–3. HEMODYNAMIC SUBSETS IN ACUTE MYOCARDIAL INFARCTION

CLINICAL SUBSET	CARDIAC INDEX ($L/min/m^2$)	PCW PRESSURE (mm Hg)	MORTALITY (%)
I. No pulmonary congestion or peripheral hypoperfusion	2.7 ± 0.5	12 ± 7	2.2
II. Isolated pulmonary congestion	2.3 ± 0.4	23 ± 5	10.1
III. Isolated peripheral hypoperfusion	1.9 ± 0.4	12 ± 5	22.4
IV. Both pulmonary congestion and hypoperfusion	1.6 ± 0.6	27 ± 8	55.5

(From Forrester JS, Diamond EG, Chatterjee K, et al: Medical therapy of acute myocardial infarction by application of hemodynamic subsets. N Engl J Med *295*:1404, 1976.)

Type and Size of Infarction

Controversy persists regarding the relation between the type of infarct and subsequent late prognosis. Some retrospective studies indicated a generally benign hospital course with a good prognosis for patients with nontransmural infarction, while others have shown that patients with nontransmural infarction have a poorer prognosis compared with those with transmural infarction. One recent prospective study (Hutter et al) showed no significant difference in immediate or late prognosis in these two subsets of patients. Sixty per cent of patients with nontransmural infarction have significant two or three vessel coronary artery obstruction, and approximately 20% of this group go on to develop an acute transmural infarction within 3 months of their initial nontransmural ischemic event.

In contrast, Roberts and coworkers have conclusively shown that the incidence of reinfarction in patients with initial nontransmural infarction is high, and cumulative mortality at 9–12 months postinfarction is similar for transmural and nontransmural subgroups. Despite the fact that high enzyme levels and clinical development of left ventricular failure are less frequent in nontransmural infarction patients, the hospital mortality and incidence of shock and arrhythmias may not differ appreciably for these patients compared with those with transmural infarction. Presumably, some of the nontransmural infarction patients are an unstable group who subsequently develop reinfarction or acute coronary insufficiency. However, when attempts are made to classify patients with myocardial infarction on the basis of initially normal versus abnormal QRS complex (previous transmural infarction, bundle branch block, or ventricular hypertrophy) and the presence or absence of *new* Q waves, it appears that the group of patients with an initially normal QRS and no Q wave evolution have a distinctly more favorable long-term prognosis than those with an abnormal QRS and no Q wave evolution (12 versus 45% mortality).

Finally, considerable controversy exists regarding the influence of the infarction site on long-term prognosis—that is, anterior versus inferior infarction. It appears that the extent of coronary artery disease and the cumulative magnitude of left ventricular dysfunction are of greater prognostic significance than is the location of the infarction.

Arrhythmias and Conduction Disturbances

The role of ventricular arrhythmias on early in-hospital mortality from acute myocardial infarction has been firmly established and will be discussed elsewhere in detail (Chapters 15, 20, 21). However, the relation between the incidence of arrhythmias post-infarction and the long-term prognosis of survivors following acute infarction remains controversial. The occurrence of ventricular ectopic activity or conduction disturbances in the late in-hospital phase of myocardial infarction is associated with a worse late prognosis. A cumulative mortality of as high as 70% at 1 year has been reported in individuals with late hospital-phase arrhythmias. Likewise, the development of high-grade atrioventricular block and new-onset trifascicular or bifascicular block in the acute phase of myocardial infarction has been associated with a high late mortality.

Poor long-term prognosis is to be expected if ventricular arrhythmias accompany significant left ventricular dysfunction, and malignant, life-threatening arrhythmias are more likely to complicate cases of left ventricular failure. Thus, it appears that cumulative myocardial damage and the severity of depressed cardiac function are the major determinants of adverse long-term prognosis.

CLINICAL APPLICATION

From the foregoing, it should be apparent that there is no unanimity regarding the utility of risk assessment following myocardial infarction, nor is there consensus that more sophisticated methods of determining prognosis have had an appreciable effect on improving or "fine-tuning" prospective care for the cardiac patient. Perhaps the most important single contribution since Killip's clinical prognostic classification has been the Forrester scheme of hemodynamic/clinical subsets (Table 11–3). Such a classification permits a more quantified approach to patient management and minimizes the likelihood of "misdiagnosis"—that is, recognition that hypotension from volume depletion can mimic peripheral hypoperfusion from intrinsically depressed cardiac function. From this standpoint, the Forrester classification facilitates an accurate assessment of *prognosis* by virtue of an improved method of *diagnosis*.

As efforts intensify to limit infarct size and salvage ischemic myocardium, it becomes clear that the ability to stratify patients with myocardial infarction on the basis of risk for reinfarction or sudden death may provide a more rational approach to the management of patients with acute ischemic heart disease, especially subgroups with postinfarct angina or late hospital-phase ventricular ectopy. Such individuals, particularly those with nontransmural infarction, may benefit from predischarge exercise testing and early cardiac catheterization, if evidence for provokable ischemia can be demonstrated.

Recent studies indicate that a limited exercise test following MI before discharge, or up to 6 weeks postinfarct, is both safe and useful. Such testing serves to identify high-risk subgroups of patients who are likely to experience another infarction or serious ventricular arrhythmia in the first year of follow-up. Since the highest percentage of deaths following discharge after myocardial infarction occurs within the first 12 months, a limited exercise test may have distinct therapeutic implications for certain patients, who may warrant aggressive management. The role of exercise testing following myocardial infarction is discussed in more detail in Chapter 26.

RECOMMENDATIONS

In the absence of signs of clinical cardiac failure or low output, assessment of prognosis requires no invasive monitoring.

In the presence of signs of clinical cardiac failure and/or low cardiac output, a Swan-Ganz thermodilution catheter insertion may clarify the patient's hemodynamic subset and permit a more quantified approach to therapy.

The assessment of cumulative myocardial damage following infarction is the critical determinant of subsequent morbidity and mortality. Quantification of regional and global ventricular wall motion and ejection fraction may facilitate a more accurate estimate of prognosis and may serve to guide subsequent diagnostic and therapeutic interventions (see Chapter 10).

The recognition and management of ventricular arrhythmias that occur late in the hospital course following myocardial infarction are of paramount importance in identifying those patients at risk of developing future coronary events and in preventing subsequent electrical complications (arrhythmogenic).

It is apparent that among survivors of acute myocardial infarction certain subgroups of patients are at higher risk of dying during the follow-up period. Following myocardial infarction, limited exercise testing before discharge from the hospital may elicit evidence for provokable myocardial ischemia or significant ventricular ectopy, both of which may presage subsequent myocardial infarction or sudden death.

SUGGESTED READING

Anderson KP, DeCamilla J, Moss AJ: Clinical significance of ventricular tachycardia (3 beats or longer) detected during ambulatory monitoring after myocardial infarction. Circulation *57*:890, 1978.

Cannom DS, Levy W and Cohen LS: The short and long-term prognosis of patients with transmural and nontransmural myocardial infarction. Am J Med *61*:452, 1976.

Forrester JS, Diamond EG, Chatterjee K, et al: Medical therapy of acute myocardial infarction by application of hemodynamic subsets. N Engl J Med *295*:1356, 1404, 1976.

Henning H, Gilpin EA, Covell JW, et al: Prognosis after acute myocardial infarction: A multivariate analysis of mortality and survival. Circulation *59*:1124, 1979.

Hutter AM Jr, Yeatman LA, Flynn T, et al: Long-term course of subendocardial myocardial infarction compared to that of anterior and inferior transmural infarction. A controlled study. Am J Cardiol *41*:398, 1978.

Killip T, Kimball JT: Treatment of myocardial infarction in a coronary care unit. Am J Cardiol *20*:457, 1967.

Kofler MN, Tabatznik B, Mower MM, et al: Prognostic significance of ventricular ectopic beats with respect to sudden death in the late post-infarction period. Circulation *47*:959, 1973.

Mahony C, Aronin N, Wagner C: The excellent short- and long-term prognosis of patients with subendocardial infarction. Am J Cardiol *41*:407, 1978.

Mahony C, Hindman MC, Aronin N, et al: Prognostic differences in subgroups of patients with electrocardiographic evidence of subendocardial or transmural myocardial infarction. The favorable outlook for patients with an initially normal QRS complex. Am J Med *69*:183, 1980.

Marmor A, Sobel BE, Roberts R: Factors presaging early recurrent myocardial infarction ("extension"). Am J Cardiol *48*:603, 1981.

Norris RM, Brandt PWT, Caughey DE, et al: A new coronary prognostic index. Lancet *1*:274, 1969.

Peel AAF, Semple T, Want I, et al: A coronary prognostic index for grading the severity of infarction. Br Heart J *24*:745, 1962.

Rigo P, Murray M, Taylor DR, et al: Hemodynamic and prognostic findings in patients with transmural and nontransmural infarction. Circulation *51*:1064, 1975.

Theroux P, Waters DD, Halphen C, et al: Prognostic value of exercise testing soon after myocardial infarction. N Engl J Med *301*:341, 1979.

Verdouw PD, Hagemeijer F, Van Dorp WG, et al: Short-term survival after acute myocardial infarction predicted by hemodynamic parameters. Circulation *52*:413, 1975.

Vismara LA, Amsterdam EA, Mason DT: Relation of ventricular arrhythmias in the late-hospital phase of acute myocardial infarction to sudden death after hospital discharge. Am J Med *59*:6, 1975.

III

INVASIVE MONITORING AND PROCEDURES IN THE CCU

12

FLOW-DIRECTED BALLOON-TIPPED PULMONARY ARTERY CATHETERS: Techniques of Insertion and Interpretation of Data; INTRAARTERIAL BLOOD PRESSURE MEASUREMENTS

William E. Boden, M.D., and
*William Kaye, M.D.**

SWAN-GANZ CATHETER

Introduction

Over the past decade, hemodynamic monitoring has advanced from the catheterization laboratory to the bedside of the CCU patient. The Swan-Ganz catheter has become a widely available clinical tool, not only in the medical center but in the community hospital as well (Fig. 12–1). Efficient and safe use of the Swan-Ganz catheter, however, presumes knowledge and expertise in the attending physician. It also requires the availability of trained nursing and paramedical personnel to manage the hemodynamic monitoring systems, including catheter care and usage and familiarity with pressure transducers and calibration technique.

This chapter will examine the usefulness of Swan-Ganz catheters (particularly as they relate to the management of patients with myocardial infarction); the physiologic information obtained from measurements of the Swan-Ganz catheter; the hemodynamic/clinical subsets that characterize left ventricular failure secondary to MI; and the indications, complications, and techniques of catheter insertion.

Clinical Utility

Important hemodynamic data can be obtained from direct measurement of the pulmonary artery pressure, the cardiac index, and determinations of oxygen saturation (based on blood samples from the pulmonary capillary bed, the pulmonary artery, and right atrium), which permit diagnostic verification of several complications of acute myocardial infarction (AMI).

*Director, Critical Care Medicine, The Miriam Hospital; Associate Professor of Surgery (Critical Care Medicine), Brown University, Providence, Rhode Island.

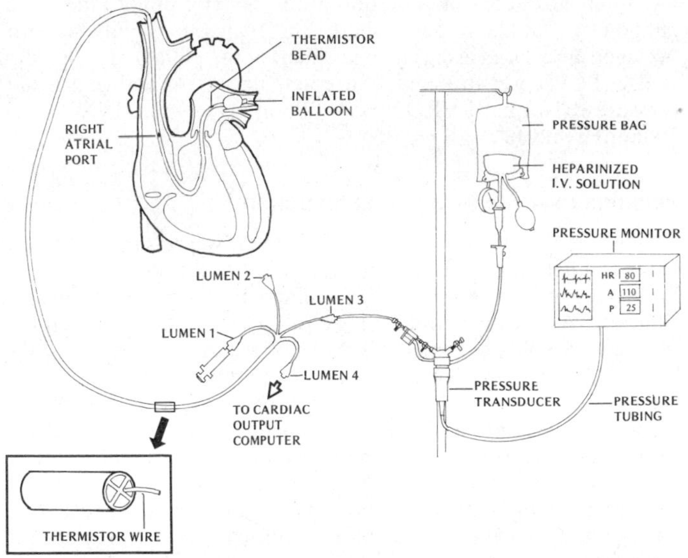

Figure 12–1. Placement and setup of a quadruple lumen pulmonary artery catheter. Lumen 1 serves for inflation of and passive deflation of the balloon. Lumen 2 terminates 30 cm from the catheter tip in the right atrium. It serves as an injector port for thermodilution cardiac output measurements and allows the measurement of right atrial pressure (CVP). Lumen 3 terminates at the tip of the catheter and allows the measurement of chamber pressures, pulmonary artery and pulmonary wedge pressures, and mixed venous sampling. Lumen 4 contains two thermistor wires, which terminate in the thermistor head 4 cm from the catheter tip.

(From Huang SH, Dasher LA, Larson CA, McCulloch CD: Coronary Care Nursing. Philadelphia, W. B. Saunders Company, 1983, p 83.)

Hemodynamic measurements obtained in patients soon after hospitalization for AMI usually reveal elevated left ventricular end-diastolic pressure (LVEDP). This increased LVEDP (or cardiac filling pressure) in the setting of AMI is usually attributable to decreased compliance (or increased "stiffness") of infarcted myocardium but also may relate to an increase in left ventricular end-diastolic volume (or myocardial fiber length). The relationship between such pressure and volume varies considerably from patient to patient and can only be inferred in any given patient.

Elevated LVEDP is transmitted to the left atrium, and, in the absence of mitral valvular disease, these elevated left-sided cardiac filling pressures are transmitted to the pulmonary capillaries, where their directional changes correlate closely with hemodynamics of the left side of the heart. Catheterization of the right heart with a

Swan-Ganz catheter and flotation of the catheter tip into the distal pulmonary capillary bed where the balloon is inflated (or "wedged") result in accurate assessment of the pulmonary capillary wedge (PCW) pressure, and, hence, left atrial (LA) and ventricular pressures. (Normal LVEDP = 3–12 mm Hg; normal PCW = 1–10 mm Hg mean.)

Findings in Acute Myocardial Infarction

Substantial elevations of LVEDP (and PCW pressure) generally indicate interstitial and, ultimately, alveolar edema, such that at PCW pressures of > 25 mm Hg, pulmonary edema is recognized clinically. Applications of Starling's Law (which states that ventricular stroke volume varies directly with ventricular end-diastolic volume) to patients with myocardial infarction indicate that increases in left ventricular volume (pressure) result in increases in cardiac output, until a plateau is attained. Further volume loading results in no additional incremental increase in myocardial function, while LV diastolic, LA, and PCW pressure rise and may result in pulmonary congestion or edema. The achievement—and subsequent maintenance—of optimal left ventricular filling pressure (or wedge pressure), therefore, is critically important to maximizing the Starling principle of peak myocardial function for patients with AMI. A PCW pressure of 15–18 mm Hg results in optimal cardiac output in most patients with AMI.

It has been recognized increasingly that hemodynamic monitoring permits the accurate identification of clinical subsets of patients with AMI. Basically, four clinical/hemodynamic subsets can be characterized by hemodynamic profiling (Table 12–1). Clearly, knowledge of the PCW pressure is crucial to identifying the appropriate hemodynamic subset and fashioning the best physiologic therapy. This is most critically apparent when one considers patients with decreased cardiac index (subsets II or IV). Individuals with depressed cardiac function may present peripheral hypoperfusion, oliguria, or an obtunded mental state (subset IV). On occasion, patients with hypovolemia may be difficult to discern clinically from subset IV, but knowledge of the PCW pressure is virtually diagnostic, since hypovolemic patients with decreased cardiac index will have *low* or normal cardiac filling pressures in contrast to patients with pump failure, who will have *high* filling pressures. Thus, many patients with low output will not need either inotropic or vasodilating agents but simply volume administration to raise their filling pressures to the optimal level.

This is also particularly true of patients with right ventricular infarction complicating left ventricular infarction, who often present initially with "hypovolemia" and decreased cardiac filling pressure (see Chapter 20). Recognition of patients in the important subgroup of "relative hypovolemia" following AMI is critically important, since management and prognosis of this subset of

Table 12–1. CLINICAL/HEMODYNAMIC SUBSETS IN AMI

	CARDIAC INDEX	PCW PRESSURE	LVSWI	SUBSET
I.	Normal	Normal	Normal	Compensated
II.	↓	↓	↓	Hypoperfusion/hypovolemia
III.	Normal	↑	Normal	Pulmonary congestion
IV.	↓	↑	↓	Pump failure

PCW = pulmonary capillary wedge
LVSWI = left ventricular stroke work index
↑ = increased
↓ = decreased

individuals who present with low cardiac output and/or shock are significantly different from that of those whose pattern of shock is secondary to massive myocardial tissue loss (true cardiogenic shock).

Indications for Swan-Ganz Catheter Use

In acute myocardial infarction

Assessment of left ventricular function

Significant systemic hypotension

Significant and persistent sinus tachycardia (≥ 110 beats/min). Such patients either may be hypovolemic or may have suffered extensive myocardial damage.

Monitoring of cardiac performance

Cardiac response to drugs

Assessment of patient prognosis

In cardiogenic shock or hypotension

In severe left ventricular failure with pulmonary edema, mitral valvular regurgitation, and/or ventricular septal rupture.

Techniques of Insertion

Insertion of the flow-directed, balloon-tipped pulmonary artery (PA) catheter (see Fig. 12–1) can be accomplished by either the percutaneous (Seldinger) technique via the femoral, subclavian, or internal jugular veins or by a cutdown of an arm vein in the antecubital fossa. The femoral approach has the advantage of easy access to a large venous conduit while the subclavian or internal jugular vein routes afford greater catheter stability once the PA line is positioned properly. Use of the antecubital vein (either a superficial or deep brachial vein) usually provides a wider margin of safety compared with other sites of entry. It is, however, the least stable of the sites.

Before commencing the procedure, the PA line insertion should be thoroughly discussed with the patient and/or family, and informed consent should be obtained. The procedure should be performed under strict sterile conditions, with cap, mask, gown,

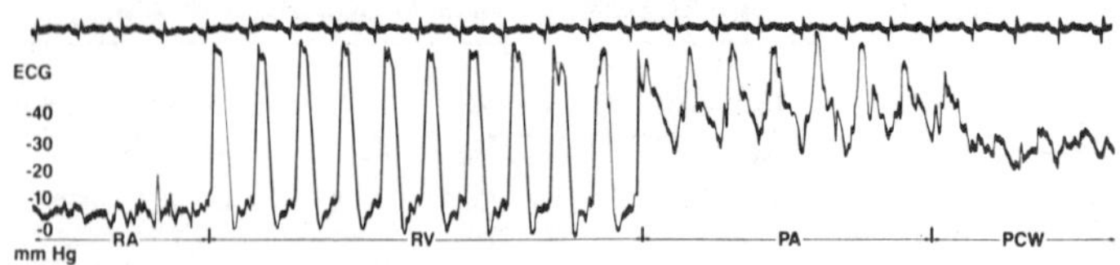

Figure 12–2. Pressure waveforms recorded as pulmonary artery catheter is advanced through right atrium (RA) and right ventricle (RV) into pulmonary artery (PA) and to wedge (PCW) position. (From Kaye W: Invasive monitoring techniques, *in* McIntyre KM, Lewis AJ (eds): Textbook of Advanced Cardiac Life Support. Copyright American Heart Association, 1981. Reproduced with permission.)

and gloves worn by the physician or operator, who should use aseptic techniques. After preparation of the appropriate skin area, use this checklist:

(1) Catheter selection—generally a 7 French (Fr) catheter is desirable because of its greater structural integrity within the vascular bed, and because of the ease of withdrawing blood samples for oxygen saturation determinations. Also, a thermodilution catheter should be selected so that cardiac output measurements can be made.
(2) Pressure transducers—it is imperative that the fluid-filled transducers be free of any air bubbles and be flushed and calibrated prior to the PA line insertion.
(3) It is important to test the integrity of the balloon before introducing it into the vein, by inflating it under water with 0.8–1.0 ml. of air, using a 1 ml. plastic tuberculin syringe.
(4) Although fluoroscopy is not absolutely necessary for introducing the PA catheter, the equipment (if portable) should be available on standby in the event it is needed. Ideally, the procedure should be employed in a "mini-catheterization" laboratory or other suitable facility that has ready access to fluoroscopy and chart recorders.

Once introduced into the vein, the catheter should be advanced through the superior vena cava to the right atrium, which is usually a distance of ~ 35 cm if the leg or the arm is used (markers are positioned at 10 cm intervals along the outer shaft of the catheter). Once the catheter tip is in the right atrium (verified by a typical right atrial [RA] pressure tracing, Fig. 12–2), 1.0–1.5 ml of air is slowly injected into the balloon port to inflate the balloon at the catheter tip. The catheter is then gently advanced through the right atrium, right ventricle (RV), and PA to the PCW position, each cardiac chamber position being verified by the characteristic pressure tracing. The recording of the PCW pressure with the balloon inflated should then be compared with the pulmonary artery end-diastolic pressure (PAEDP) with balloon deflated. In the majority of patients, the value of PAEDP is within 1–2 mm Hg of that of the PCW pressure; thus, continuous monitoring of the PAEDP is practical and safe, particularly in view of the fact that repeated balloon inflations can lead to balloon rupture or, more significantly, to a situation in which the catheter becomes "wedged" in the capillary position. Such prolonged wedging of the catheter has been reported to produce pulmonary infarction.

After passage of the catheter into the PCW position, the balloon should be deflated. Prior to each inflation of the balloon, the catheter should be aspirated to assure that air is not trapped in the balloon or that blood is not returned (indicating a rupture of the balloon). When inflating the balloon for the purpose of recording PCW pressure, care should be taken to add air slowly until visual inspection of the PA pressure tracing changes to the PCW pressure configuration. Frequent monitoring of the catheter tip is necessary to prevent its inadvertent migration into the "wedged" position. A chest radiograph should be made after the procedure to verify the catheter position. Finally, the catheter should be anchored firmly to the skin at its entry site with stay sutures, to prevent catheter malposition. To maintain catheter patency, it is recommended that a constant infusion through the catheter lumen be maintained at all times and that small amounts of heparin be added to the infusate.

In about 10–15% of patients, the Swan-Ganz catheter cannot be advanced beyond the right ventricular outflow tract. Usually these patients have marked pulmonary hypertension and right ventricular enlargement, resulting in low cardiac output. Attempts to position the Swan-Ganz catheter in the PA are often fruitless, even with fluoroscopic guidance.

Complications of Hemodynamic Monitoring

Serious ventricular arrhythmias during passage of the catheter through the RV. This can be minimized by the prophylactic administration of intravenous lidocaine before the PA catheter is passed through the RV.

Pulmonary infarction due to prolonged wedging of the catheter. This can be minimized by using the PAEDP as a guide to LV filling pressures, inflating the balloon only intermittently, flushing the catheter at regular intervals, and checking the position of the catheter tip. All CCU personnel should be familiar with the appearance of the PCW pressure, so that inadvertent migration of the catheter into the wedged position can be readily detected.

Infection. Attention paid to aseptic technique should lessen the incidence of infection. Generally, as with any indwelling catheter, the incidence of infection is higher when the line remains in place longer than 48–72 hours.

Data

Figure 12–2 illustrates a typical sequence of characteristic cardiac chamber pressures that is obtained when a Swan-Ganz catheter is inserted into the right heart.

INTRAARTERIAL BLOOD PRESSURE MEASUREMENT

Introduction

Arterial cannulation for continuous intraarterial blood pressure monitoring is easily and rapidly accomplished at the bedside. However, operators must be skilled in the appropriate technique; they must be familiar with both the catheter and transducer system in order to eliminate air bubbles and prevent clots and contamination; they must correctly calibrate the system and avoid artifacts.

For the patient in shock with elevated systemic vascular resistance, a significant discrepancy may be registered between pressure obtained by auscultation and palpation methods and pressure obtained by the direct intraarterial pressure method. The intraarterial pressure may be much higher than the pressure recorded with the sphygmomanometer. Failure to recognize the fact that low cuff pressure does not necessarily indicate arterial hypotension may lead to dangerous errors in therapy; continuous intraarterial pressure monitoring eliminates this pitfall.

In addition, any patient who requires titrated intravenous vasopressors or vasodilators for improved hemodynamics must have intraarterial pressure continuously recorded. Continuous intraarterial pressure monitoring allows the physician to titrate the dosage of such drugs according to the blood pressure response and permits the accurate detection of sudden changes in pressure that may follow the use of vasodilators or sympathomimetic amines.

Site of Cannulation

The *radial artery* is the most commonly used site for cannulation, is generally safe, and is free from potential complications when careful attention is directed to demonstrating adequate ulnar collateral flow prior to cannulation. In the event of thrombosis of the radial artery at the catheter site, ischemic injury of the hand is rare if there is adequate ulnar collateral flow. The *axillary artery* is a large artery with excellent collateral flow, indicative of the fact that thrombosis would not lead to any serious sequelae. However, embolism of air or thrombus (which may form at the catheter tip) can produce ischemic injury to the brain or the hand. For this reason, the axillary artery is not a preferred site for arterial cannulation. The *femoral artery* is another large artery frequently

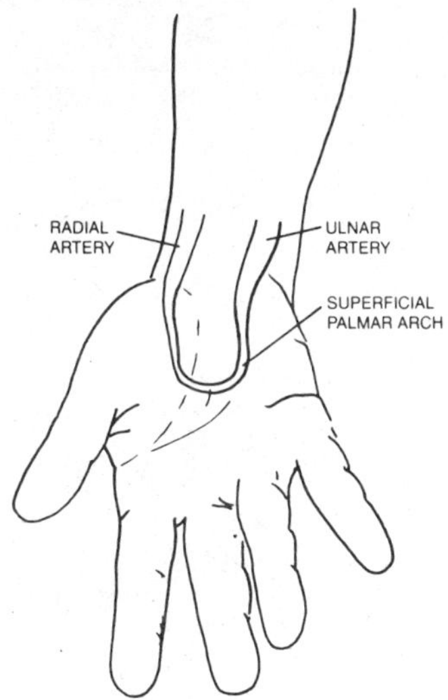

Figure 12–3. Anatomy of radial and ulnar arteries at wrist and superficial palmar arch. (From Kaye W: Invasive monitoring techniques, *in* McIntyre KM, Lewis AJ (eds): Textbook of Advanced Cardiac Life Support. Copyright American Heart Association, 1981. Reproduced with permission.)

used for monitoring pressures, but it should be avoided in the presence of occlusive arterial disease of the lower extremity.

Preparation for Radial Artery Cannulation

Prior to cannulation of the radial artery, it is necessary to document adequacy of ulnar collateral flow via the superficial palmar arch (Fig. 12–3). The superficial palmar arch is formed from the continuation of the ulnar artery into the hand. Twelve per cent of hands either have poor collateral flow or have an incomplete palmar arch with no collateral circulation whatever. The modified Allen test is useful for determining the presence of collateral circulation:

1. If the patient's hands are not warm, they should be immersed in warm water to make pulsations more easily demonstrable.

2. Have the patient open and close the hand, held overhead or out in front, several times to decrease relative blood flow, then grasp the tightly clenched fist. (If the patient is unconscious or under anesthesia, clench the fist passively for him or her.)

3. Occlude both the radial and the ulnar arteries, then have the patient lower and open the hand. When the hand is open, it should be relaxed; hyperextension of the wrist or hand should be avoided since this increases the tension of the palmar fascia, which in turn compresses arterial microcirculation. Failure to relax the hand, or hyperextending the hand at the wrist, may cause a falsely abnormal Allen test.

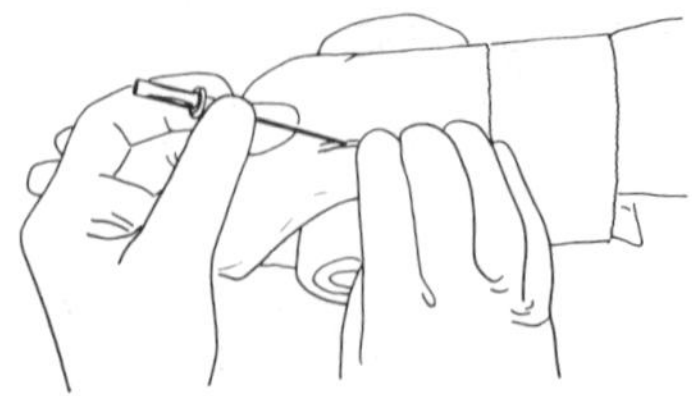

Figure 12–4. Cannulation of radial artery. (From Kaye W: Invasive monitoring techniques, *in* McIntyre KM, Lewis AJ (eds): Textbook of Advanced Cardiac Life Support. Copyright American Heart Association, 1981. Reproduced with permission.)

4. Release the pressure over the ulnar artery only and observe the open hand for return of color; color return within 6 seconds indicates patency of the ulnar artery and an intact arch. Delay of color return from 7 to 15 seconds indicates that ulnar artery filling is slow. Persistent blanching for up to 15 seconds or more indicates an incomplete ulnar arch. Hands with delayed or absent return of color upon release of ulnar compression (positive Allen test) should not be used for radial artery cannulation.

Equipment Required

20 gauge Teflon catheter-over-needle with nontapered shaft, 1¼ to 2″ (3.2 to 5.1 cm) in length

Short armboard and roll of gauze

Povidone-iodine solution

1% lidocaine without epinephrine and 3 ml syringe with 25 gauge needle

Sterile gloves and sterile drapes (face mask and hair cover for optimal asepsis)

Fluid-filled connecting tubing to transducer

Technique (Fig. 12–4)

The patient's hand should be dorsiflexed approximately 60° at the wrist.

Locate the radial artery proximal to the head of the radius.

Cleanse the area with povidone-iodine solution.

Wear sterile gloves and drape the area with sterile towels.

Infiltrate the overlying skin with 1% lidocaine without epinephrine

While palpating the artery: Insert the catheter-needle device at about a 30° angle and advance the catheter and needle stylet into the artery until blood appears in the hub of the needle.

While holding the stylet in the fixed position, advance the catheter over the stylet into the artery until only the hub is visible.

Remove the inner stylet and attach the hub of the catheter to connecting tubing.

Tie the catheter securely in place.

Fix the wrist in neutral position to a board.

Apply povidone-iodine ointment to the skin at the insertion site and cover with a sterile dressing.

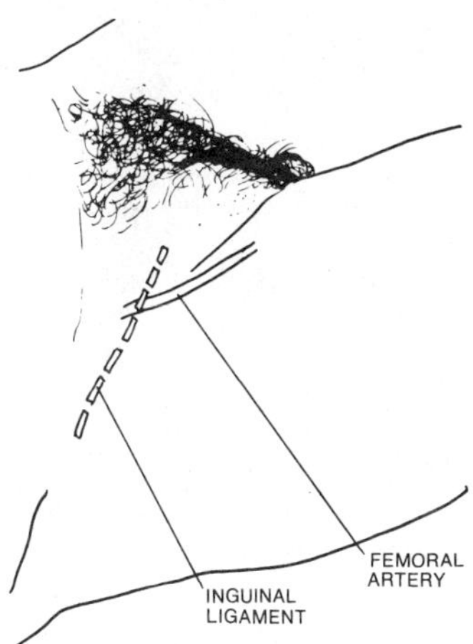

Figure 12–5. Anatomy of femoral artery. (From Kaye W: Invasive monitoring techniques, *in* McIntyre KM, Lewis AJ (eds): Textbook of Advanced Cardiac Life Support. Copyright American Heart Association, 1981. Reproduced with permission.)

Cannulation of the Femoral Artery (Fig. 12–5)

The site for cannulation of the femoral artery should be approximately 2 cm below the inguinal ligament or near the inguinal fold.

Equipment Required

19 or 20 gauge Teflon catheter, 16 cm long

Flexible guidewire small enough to pass through the catheter and needle

20 gauge needle, 5 cm in length

Other equipment (Seldinger or Potts needle) as for any arterial cannulation

Technique (Fig. 12–6)

Identify the femoral artery and choose a site approximately 2 cm below the inguinal ligament or near the inguinal fold.

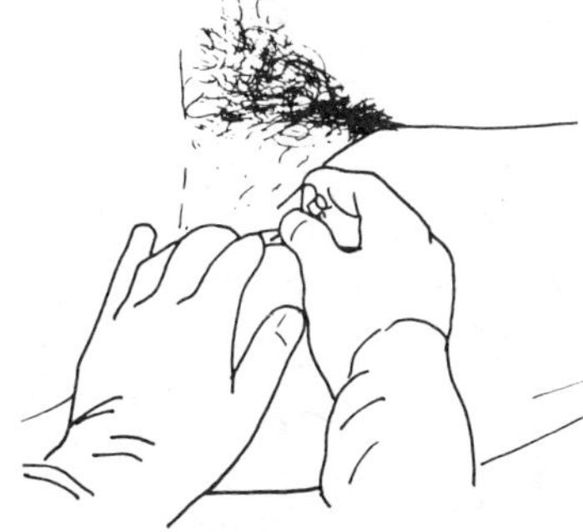

Figure 12–6. Cannulation of femoral artery. (From Kaye W: Invasive monitoring techniques, *in* McIntyre KM, Lewis AJ (eds): Textbook of Advanced Cardiac Life Support. Copyright American Heart Association, 1981. Reproduced with permission.)

Shave the groin and cleanse the skin with povidone-iodine.

Wear sterile gloves, mask, and hair cover.

Cover the area around the insertion site with sterile drapes.

Place the fingers of one hand along the course of the femoral artery beyond the inguinal ligament.

Infiltrate the overlying skin with 1% lidocaine without epinephrine.

Puncture the skin and, using the Seldinger technique, aim the needle directly at the arterial pulsation and artery at about a 45° angle. Pass the wire through the needle into the artery and then remove the needle. Do not insert the wire against resistance.

No syringe is connected to the Seldinger needle during withdrawal. A large (2–5 cm arc), pulsating stream of blood should emerge from the end of the needle when its tip is completely within the lumen of the arterial vessel.

Insert the catheter over the wire, then remove the wire from the catheter and attach the connecting tubing to the end of the catheter.

Suture the catheter in place with 3–0 silk.

Cover the insertion site with povidone-iodine ointment and a sterile dressing.

Cannulation of the Axillary Artery

The axillary artery is a continuation of the subclavian artery as it leaves the root of the neck to enter the axilla at the lateral border of the first rib. Because of the extensive collateral circulation that exists between the thyrocervical trunk of the subclavian artery and the subscapular artery (which is a branch of the distal axillary artery), ligation or thrombosis of the axillary artery usually will not lead to compromise of flow to the distal arm or forearm. The axillary artery is a large artery, almost the size of the femoral artery.

Equipment Required

For insertion with the Seldinger technique, a 19 or 20 gauge Teflon catheter (16 cm long), a flexible guidewire that fits both needle and catheter, and a 20 gauge needle (5 cm long) or a 20 gauge catheter-over-needle device (with a catheter at least 6.4 cm long) as needed

Povidone-iodine solution

1% lidocaine without epinephrine and a 3 mm syringe with a 25 gauge needle

Sterile gloves and drapes, face mask, and hair cover

Fluid-filled connecting tubing to transducer

Technique

Immobilize the arm, with the arm externally rotated and hyperabducted more than 90° from the patient's body.

Stand at the patient's side, either above or below the abducted arm.

Locate the artery within the axilla.

Shave and cleanse the skin with povidone-iodine solution.

Wear sterile gloves, mask, and hair cover; drape the area with sterile towels.

Infiltrate the skin with 1% lidocaine without epinephrine.

Insert the needle into the artery as high as possible within the axilla.

If the Seldinger technique is used, pass the wire through the needle into the artery and remove the needle once free arterial flow is obtained.

Complications of Arterial Cannulation

Arterial occlusive disease, diabetes mellitus, Raynaud's disease, hypothermia, autoimmune diseases with vasculitis, and excessive and prolonged pressure on the artery to control bleeding following catheter removal predispose to thrombosis and the ischemic sequelae of thrombosis. With intermittent flushing, the incidence of thrombosis is increased. A continuous flush system should be used to insure catheter patency, prevent thrombosis, and minimize the incidence of embolism. The arterial line should be continuously flushed with a heparinized (10,000 units/1000 ml 5% dextrose solution) infusate. With a continuous flush system one can also monitor catheter patency. By opening the flush valve and then rapidly closing it, a square wave is generated on the arterial wave form that indicates no clot or bubbles are present in the system. If clots, bubbles, or loose connections are present, the square wave response will be damped significantly.

Embolism

Embolism is more common when intermittent flushing of the catheter is performed by hand. A continuous flush system that eliminates the need for intermittent flushing minimizes this problem. Embolism may occur from small clots that form around the tip of the catheter or by air and particulate matter introduced into the system.

Hemorrhage

Rapid exsanguination of the patient may follow any disconnection of the arterial line between the patient and the transducer, unless this event is promptly recognized. A coagulopathy, either caused by anticoagulation or a disease process, increases the incidence of hemorrhage from the puncture site. Hypertension may also increase the incidence of bleeding. A hematoma following removal of the arterial catheter is common.

Infection

The most obvious risk factor for catheter-related infection appears to be the length of time the catheter resides in the vessel; most infections are caused by arterial catheters left in place for more than 72 hours. Arterial catheters inserted by cutdown involve an increased incidence of infection compared with catheters inserted percutaneously.

To minimize the possibility of infection, the catheter must be inserted using strict aseptic technique. Percutaneous insertion rather than insertion by cut-down is preferred. The insertion site must be aseptically inspected and redressed at least once every 48 hours. The catheter should be removed after 72 hours or sooner if signs of inflammation at the insertion site are seen.

Neurologic Complications

During attempts at axillary arterial puncture, direct injury to the cords of the brachial plexus may occur, or an axillary sheath hematoma may lead to nerve compression and injury. The axillary artery, therefore, should not be used for intraarterial monitoring in patients with bleeding diatheses.

Arteriovenous Fistula

A fistula between the femoral artery and the femoral vein may be produced, especially when larger catheters such as those employed during cardiac catheterization and angiography are used.

CARE OF THE CATHETER, TRANSDUCER, AND ELECTRONIC MONITOR

To ensure that pressures recorded from the intraarterial cannulae are accurate, great care must be exercised with the entire system. Artifacts can be minimized by observing the following procedures:

Allow the transducer and amplifier to warm up for at least 10 minutes before starting to zero and calibrate the system.

Mechanically zero the transducer to the level of the patient's right atrium. The level of the right atrium or the phlebostatic axis in the supine patient is the midpoint of a line drawn from the outermost point of the sternum to the outermost point of the posterior chest, or the midaxillary line. Although it may not be possible accurately to compare absolute values from patient to patient using the phlebostatic axis, at least the patient can serve as his or her own control, and changes in pressures will have an accurate reference point. The phlebostatic axis should be marked with indelible ink on each patient.

Purge all air from the pressure system.

Check all fittings for tightness.

Electrically zero and calibrate the system with the mercury manometer or a water column.

Use stiff, noncompliant extension tubing of shortest possible length and avoid use of more than one stopcock between catheter and transducer.

Avoid draining blood samples the full length of the tubing system.

Maintain the catheter so that clotting does not occur.

Recheck the mechanical and electrical zero position and recalibrate the system, if necessary, when the level of the patient is changed.

Avoid making adjustments to the amplifier except at the time of calibration.

Check the zero setting (both electrically and mechanically) and calibration at least once per shift.

MEASURES TO PREVENT TRANSDUCER-RELATED *INFECTION*

The transducer should be gas sterilized. As an alternative, disposable domes may be used.

Use aseptic technique when transducers are calibrated and set up for use.

Employ a simple arrangement of tubing and stopcocks with disposable components.

Adhere to aseptic technique during in-use manipulation.

Blood samples can be drawn through a stopcock placed near the catheter. Never disconnect tubing for blood drawing.

Treat stopcocks as a sterile field and keep covered with a sterile cap.

Do not allow blood to remain in the stopcock port.

Change transducers, connecting tubing, and flushing fluid every 48 hours if possible.

REFERENCES

Bageant RA: Variations in arterial blood gas analysis due to sampling techniques. Resp. Care *20*:565, 1975.

Forrester JS, Diamond G, Chatterjee K, et al: Medical therapy of acute myocardial infarction by application of hemodynamic subsets. N Engl J Med *295*:1356, 1404, 1976.

Kaye W: Invasive monitoring techniques, *in* Textbook of Advanced Cardiac Life Support. New York, American Heart Association, XIII, 1–32, 1981.

Kemp GL: Questions and answers: Arterial blood samplers should be stored on ice for gas analysis. JAMA *223*:696, 1973.

Petty TL, Bigelow DB, Levine BE: The simplicity and safety of arterial puncture. JAMA *195*:693, 1966.

Swan HJC, Ganz W, Forrester JS, et al: Catheterization of the heart in man with the use of flow-directed balloon-tipped catheter. N Engl J Med *283*:447, 1970.

13

TEMPORARY TRANSVENOUS CARDIAC PACEMAKERS

*William Kaye, M.D.**

A cardiac pacemaker delivers an electrical stimulus to the heart, causing depolarization and cardiac contraction. Usually temporary pacing is accomplished by passing a pacemaker wire transvenously into the heart where it stimulates the endocardium.

The cardiac pacing wire may be placed in the right atrium or the ventricle. Atrioventricular sequential pacing is also employed when a wire is placed concomitantly in both the right atrium and the right ventricle; the atrium and the ventricle are sequentially paced, mimicking the normal temporal sequence of cardiac contraction. Both atrial pacing in the presence of intact atrioventricular conduction and atrioventricular sequential pacing provide an atrial "kick" that augments ventricular stroke volume. In contrast, the stroke volume with ventricular pacing may be significantly less in the absence of the atrial contribution to ventricular filling. However, atrial pacing is difficult, since the pacing electrode tends to become easily dislodged, with resultant loss of capture. Atrial pacing may be employed for overdrive suppression of supraventricular tachyarrhythmias.

Ventricular pacing is generally easier and more reliable. In the presence of atrioventricular conduction disturbances, either ventricular pacing or atrioventricular sequential pacing must be employed. Ventricular pacing may be employed for overdrive suppression of refractory ventricular tachyarrhythmias.

EQUIPMENT

An external pacemaker system has two basic components: an *external pulse generator* and a *pacing electrode*. Characteristics of an external pulse generator include

(1) Output with variable amplitude (in milliamperes [mA]), which allows definition of the threshold for ventricular capture and the ability to alter pacemaker output if the threshold changes;

(2) Fixed and demand modes of pacing. In the fixed mode, the pulse generator emits stimuli at regular intervals, regardless of cardiac activity. In the demand mode, a pacemaker rate is selected;

---

*Director, Critical Care Medicine, The Miraim Hospital; Associate Professor of Surgery (Critical Care Medicine), Brown University, Providence, Rhode Island.

if the intrinsic heart rate exceeds the rate of the pacemaker, the pacemaker generator will be inhibited. However, if the intrinsic heart rate falls below the predetermined rate on the external pulse generator, the pacemaker will generate an impulse;

(3) Variable rate setting. The rate setting determines the rate that the pacemaker will generate impulses in both the fixed and demand modes; and

(4) Indicators that show each pacemaker-generated impulse, as well as intrinsic heart beats that occur when the pacer is inhibited.

Two types of pacing electrodes are available. A *bipolar pacing electrode catheter* is most commonly used. Both electrodes of a bipolar catheter are in contact with the endocardial surface of the heart; the catheter usually requires fewer repositionings to maintain its optimal capturing function. In contrast, in a *unipolar catheter* only the cathode is in contact with the heart, with a subcutanuous ground lead (anode) placed some distance from the heart. Compared with a bipolar electrode, the unipolar lead may have a lower pacing threshold and may provide more reliable demand function in the presence of small intracardiac signals.

When ventricular capture cannot be accomplished with a bipolar lead, pacemaker function may be restored by converting to a unipolar system. The proximal (anode) electrode from the bipolar pacemaker catheter is disconnected from the pacemaker generator and a metal suture and wire are inserted subcutaneously into the chest wall; this wire is connected to the anode of the pulse generator to complete the electrical circuit.

INDICATIONS FOR THE EMERGENCY CARDIAC PACEMAKER

Emergency cardiac pacing is indicated for treatment of symptomatic bradyarrhythmias, for prophylaxis of conduction disturbances that occur during acute myocardial infarction, and for control of supraventricular and ventricular tachyarrhythmias by overdrive suppression.

Symptomatic Bradyarrhythmias. Since cardiac output is the product of heart rate and stroke volume, it is axiomatic that the stroke volume must increase to maintain cardiac output if the heart rate slows appreciably. If cardiac output falls, systemic vascular resistance must rise in order to maintain blood pressure. Marked slowing of the ventricular rate upon the development of high-grade AV block may be followed by failure of these compensatory mechanisms, especially in individuals who have abnormal hearts. This failure of compensatory adjustments may lead to symptoms of hypoperfusion and hypotension (including light-headedness, syncope, and seizures), pulmonary congestion, and increased myocardial ischemia. Such patients are best managed with a cardiac pacemaker to maintain ventricular rate and to permit the use of antiarrhythmic drugs to suppress atrial or ventricular tachyarrhythmias that may occur.

Prophylactic Pacing and Acute Myocardial Infarction. In acute *inferior* myocardial infarction, the new development of Mobitz type I second-degree atrioventricular (AV) block is *generally not* an indication for pacemaker insertion. However, if the ventricular rate is slow enough to produce the symptoms (hypotension and hypoperfusion) described earlier that are refractory to atropine, then a cardiac pacemaker is indicated. In contrast, the development of Mobitz type II second-degree heart block in inferior wall myocardial infarction *is* indication for a temporary pacemaker, even though the ventricular rate is not producing symptoms, since complete (third-degree) AV block may follow abruptly.

With *anterior* myocardial infarction, the new onset of second-degree AV block (Mobitz type *I* or Mobitz type *II*) *is* an indication for insertion of a stand-by demand pacemaker, since third-degree AV block with an unstable ventricular subsidiary pacemaker may occur abruptly without any premonitory signs. The occurrence of new bifascicular block (right bundle branch block with either left anterior hemiblock or left posterior hemiblock) or new bilateral bundle branch block (trifascicular block or alternating bundle branch block) is another indication for prophylactic pacing in the setting of an acute myocardial infarction. These conduction abnormalities are often (and unpredictably) followed by complete AV block. Following the new onset of isolated right or left bundle branch block, some physicians prefer to insert a temporary pacemaker, while others prefer only to monitor the patient closely.

Overdrive Pacing for Atrial or Ventricular Tachyarrhythmias. Atrial flutter and supraventricular tachycardia may be converted to normal sinus rhythm by rapid atrial pacing. Rapid pacing of the atrium however, is not without significant hazard; it is possible for the pacing catheter to be displaced into the right ventricle with capture of the ventricle, resulting in ventricular fibrillation. Overdrive pacing of the ventricle may be effective in the treatment of refractory ventricular arrhythmias. Ventricular arrhythmias may be prevented by acceleration of the heart rate; however, the rate of overdrive does not have to exceed the rate of the ectopic mechanism and need only be faster than the normal sinus pacemaker to be effective in interrupting a reentrant-type focus. (See Chapter 15.)

GENERAL PRINCIPLES FOR PACEMAKER CATHETER INSERTION

Aseptic Technique. It is vital to observe strict aseptic technique during pacemaker insertion, since the catheter may remain in the patient for several days. To minimize infection, the area of insertion must be carefully prepared with povidone-iodine solution; the operator and assistant must be fully gowned and wear hair covers, face masks, and sterile gloves. The area around the insertion site must be covered with sterile drapes large enough to prevent contamination of the long catheter. After positioning of the pacemaker catheter, the insertion site should be covered with a sterile dressing and should be inspected, using sterile techniques, for signs of phlebitis or local infection for at least 48 hours.

During emergency pacemaker insertion, the ECG should be continuously monitored. An IV catheter must be in place, and resuscitation equipment, including a defibrillator and essential cardiac drugs, should be immediately available at the bedside.

Monitoring Catheter Tip Location. The transvenous catheter may be inserted under fluoroscopic guidance or blindly. The location of the intracardiac catheter during blind insertion is determined either by recording the intracardiac electrogram from the catheter tip (the preferred method), or by using the pacemaker spike and evidence for ventricular capture. If fluoroscopy is used (either at the bedside or in the catheterization or angiography suite), the fluoroscopy image intensifier tube should be turned on, centered over the heart, and tested for adequate imaging before the procedure begins. It is, of course, essential that the operator be familiar with operation of the fluoroscopy equipment and good fluoroscopy technique.

To monitor the intracardiac electrogram from the catheter tip during insertion, the limb leads of an ECG machine, which must be properly grounded with less than 10 microamps of current leakage, are attached to the patient. The V lead is attached to the wire from the distal electrode of the pacing catheter, using an electrically safe adaptor, and the electrogram from the V lead is recorded (Fig. 13–1). As the catheter is advanced into the right atrium, large negative P waves and small QRS complexes are recorded. In the low right atrium, and as the catheter is advanced into the right ventricle, P waves become positive, and the QRS complex becomes more prominent than the P waves. When the catheter electrode tip touches the endocardial surface of the right ventricle, ST segment elevation (transient injury current) is seen, indicating that the catheter should be in proper position for ventricular pacing.

In emergency situations requiring immediate pacemaker insertion (e.g., the asystolic cardiac arrest patient), blind insertion of the pacing catheter via the percutaneous route, or the transthoracic approach, may be attempted. To use evidence of ventricular capture for determining the location of the intracardiac catheter, the pacemaker electrodes are attached to the pulse generator, and the rate of the generator is set at a level above the patient's intrinsic heart rate, with the amplitude or output set at maximum. While recording a surface ECG, the pacemaker is advanced into the

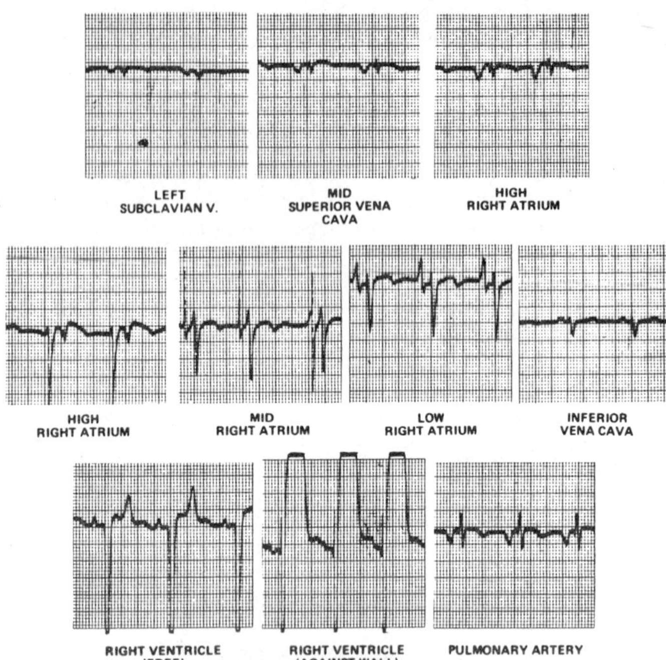

Figure 13–1. Electrocardiographic monitoring of catheter tip location. (Adapted from Bing OHL, McDowell JW, Hantman J, et al: Pacemaker placement by electrocardiographic monitoring. N Engl J Med 287:651, 1972.)

heart. Contact with the endocardium of the desired chamber (right atrium or right ventricle) is recognized as capture by the pacemaker on the surface ECG.

Determination of Pacing Threshold. Once the pacemaker catheter is in proper position, the threshold of stimulation must be determined. The amplitude of the output signal is gradually decreased until capture is lost; this is the *pacing threshold.* A low pacing threshold of less than 1.0 mA indicates that the electrode is in optimal contact with the endocardium. If the pacing threshold is high and the need for pacing is not urgent, the catheter may be repositioned until a lower pacing threshold is obtained. However, if the need for pacing is urgent, the output is turned as high as necessary to achieve atrioventricular capture. If the threshold is low, the *maintenance current* for pacing should be set at 2–3 times the threshold current. It is helpful also to instruct the patient, if awake, to take deep breaths, cough, and shift position in bed to assess the stability of the pacing site and the maintenance of capture.

Care should be exercised when turning off the pacemaker, since the patient's previous rhythm may not return promptly after even a brief period of pacing.

Demand Mode. The pulse generator should be set in the demand mode to avoid competition between the artificial pacemaker and spontaneous rhythm, which may lead to ventricular fibrillation.

Chest Radiograph. A chest radiograph must be obtained as soon as pacemaker insertion is accomplished, to verify proper position and to exclude the presence of pneumothorax (if the catheter was inserted via the internal jugular or subclavian veins). If a lateral film is taken, the catheter tip should point anteriorly, which indicates that the catheter tip is in the right ventricle; the catheter tip pointing posteriorly may indicate that the tip is in the coronary sinus or has perforated the ventricle.

CHOICE OF PACEMAKER SITE AND CATHETER FOR INSERTION

A pacemaker catheter may be inserted percutaneously via the *internal jugular, subclavian, femoral,* or *antecubital veins,* or by cut-down through a *median antecubital vein.*

A catheter inserted through the median antecubital vein of the arm is commonly displaced with arm movement; this results in loss of pacing, extrusion of the catheter from the ventricle, or myocardial perforation. In addition, sepsis and phlebitis may be more common at this site.

Percutaneous cannulation of either the internal jugular or subclavian vein is easily performed, and insertion of a pacemaker via these routes generally provides stable pacing while at the same time permitting full arm motion, and limited ambulatory activities. However, the potential complications of internal jugular and subclavian venipuncture include pneumothorax, carotid or subclavian artery puncture, and brachial plexus injury.

Insertion of a balloon-tipped catheter percutaneously into the femoral vein is also simple and rapid, except that on occasion stiffer catheters may be required because soft catheters may form angles or loops during passage up the inferior vena cava or may float away from endocardial contact. Finally, rapid flexion of the cannulated leg at the hip after pacemaker insertion may lead to forward propulsion of the catheter into the right ventricle, producing loss of capture or perforation. Phlebitis and thromboembolism occur rarely but must be considered as potential complications.

Two types of pacemaker catheters are commonly employed: *balloon-tipped catheters* and *regular pacing catheters.* A balloon-tipped catheter, either 3 or 5 French (Fr), is generally preferred for a blind insertion, whereas regular pacing catheters (4–7 Fr) are generally inserted under fluoroscopic guidance.

Blind Catheter Insertion from Subclavian, Internal Jugular, or Brachial Vein

Equipment Required

A 3 or 5 Fr balloon-tipped bipolar pacing catheter

Pulse generator and connecting cable

Electrically safe ECG machine with adaptor to connect distal catheter electrode to V lead

Equipment for percutaneous catheter sheath insertion (cutdown equipment for brachial insertion, if necessary)

Sterile drapes, gown, gloves, hair covers, masks; material for cleansing insertion site

Technique

Cleanse the insertion site and drape the patient in a sterile manner.

Infiltrate the skin with lidocaine.

Test the balloon before insertion.

Attach limb leads of ECG machine to patient.

Insert catheter into the vein, either through percutaneous catheter sheath or via cutdown.

Attach V lead of ECG machine to distal electrode terminal. Inflate the balloon when the catheter is high in the right atrium.

Advance the catheter, following the intracavitary electrocardiogram.

Deflate the balloon when the catheter passes into the right ventricle.

Insert the catheter farther until the ST segment elevation is seen on the ECG, indicating contact with the right ventricular endocardium.

Disconnect the V lead from the pacemaker catheter and attach the connecting cable from the pulse generator to the electrode terminals.

Document ventricular capture and the pacing threshold while recording a surface ECG.

Set the generator output two to three times above threshold in the demand mode at the desired rate.

Secure the catheter in place and cover the insertion site.

Obtain a chest radiograph, including a lateral view, to observe catheter position and to detect pneumothorax or other complications related to insertion.

Immobilize the arm if the catheter is inserted via the brachial vein.

Blind Catheter Insertion from the Femoral Vein

Equipment Required

A 5 Fr balloon-tipped bipolar pacing catheter

Other equipment listed in preceding section

Technique

Shave and cleanse the groin and drape in a sterile manner.

Infiltrate the skin with lidocaine.

Attach ECG limb leads to the patient.

Insert the catheter through the sheath into the vein.

If a balloon-tipped catheter is used, inflate the balloon after the catheter has been inserted approximately 15 cm.

Attach the V lead from the ECG machine to the distal electrode terminal.

Advance the catheter, using the intracavitary ECG to determine catheter tip location. Several passage attempts may be necessary to obtain proper ventricular capture.

Deflate the balloon of a balloon catheter when the catheter crosses the tricuspid valve. Insert the catheter until ST elevation is seen on the electrocardiogram recorded from the catheter tip.

When the catheter is positioned in the right ventricle, follow the technique previously described.

COMPLICATIONS OF CARDIAC PACING

Thrombophlebitis and Pulmonary Emboli. Phlebitis and/or thrombosis of *any* vein may develop after a catheter is inserted, but pulmonary embolism from a temporary transvenous pacemaker is rare.

Sepsis. A local infection at the insertion site and/or bacteremia may follow insertion of a pacing catheter under emergency conditions with less than optimal asepsis and may follow frequent manipulations of repositioning the catheter. The incidence of local and systemic infection increases as a function of the duration of time the pacing catheter is left in place. Inspection and care and redressing of the insertion site, using aseptic technique, must be performed at least once every 48 hours.

Perforation of the Right Ventricle. Perforation of the right ventricle is uncommon but usually occurs without sequelae. Signs of ventricular perforation include loss of pacing (capture); synchronous diaphragmatic, intercostal, or abdominal contraction at the same rate as the pacemaker; or the development of a pericardial friction rub. Electrocardiographic changes suggestive of electrode perforation include a change in the frontal plane vector of the pacemaker artifact and a change in the QRS complex from the usual left bundle branch block pattern seen with right ventricular endocardial pacemakers to a right bundle branch block pattern. Cardiac tamponade following perforation of the right ventricle is rare; the only treatment usually required is to withdraw the catheter into the right ventricle until normal sensing and capture reappear. Myocardial perforation is more common with stiff catheters and when the catheter is inserted from the arm or femoral vein. Diaphragmatic stimulation may indicate myocardial perforation, although it may also occur without perforation.

Pacemaker Generator Failure. Generator failure includes failure of sensing, oversensing, and failure of pacing. Sensing failure of a demand pacemaker is most commonly due to a low amplitude QRS signal, especially with a bipolar catheter; the signal may be increased either by repositioning the catheter or by converting to a unipolar system. A failing battery also may lead to loss of sensing.

Oversensing may be due to undesirable signals originating either from the patient (skeletal muscle contractions, large P or T waves, loose pacemaker connections, or intermittent separation of a fractured wire) or from extraneous sources (electromagnetic fields, stray electrical currents, and manipulation of the connecting cable).

Failure of pacing with loss of pacing artifact may be due either to fracture of the catheter tip or failure of the generator. Failure of pacing with persistence of the pacing artifact indicates malposition of the catheter or excessive threshold, battery depletion with enough current present to generate an artifact but not enough to depolarize the heart, or a break in the electrode insulation that reduces the output of the catheter tip.

Cardiac Arrhythmias Induced by Pacemakers. Arrhythmias may occur during insertion and during subsequent pacing. Both endocardial irritation and competition may induce ventricular fibrillation, especially in an ischemic heart characterized by a lower fibrillation threshold. The risk of pacemaker-induced arrhythmias is also increased in the presence of metabolic acidosis, hypoxemia, excessive sympathetic activity, and digitalis excess.

Pacemaker-Induced Heart Sounds. A pacemaker may induce presystolic clicks (diaphragmatic or costal muscle stimulation), systolic clicks and murmurs (movement of the catheter within the right ventricle or catheter-induced tricuspid insufficiency), and friction rubs (contact of the catheter with the endocardium or following myocardial perforation).

Knotting of the Catheter. A flexible pacing catheter may knot upon itself or around other intracardiac catheters.

ST and T Wave Abnormalities Following Cessation of Pacing. T wave inversion and ST segment depression may occur on the unpaced electrocardiogram subsequent to ventricular pacing. These changes may persist for a variable length of time after termination of pacing and may be difficult to distinguish from ischemia.

REFERENCES

Bing OH, McDowell JW, Hantman J et al: Pacemaker placement by electrocardiographic monitoring N Engl J Med *287*:651, 1972.

Cheng FI: Percutaneous transfemoral venous cardiac pacing. A simple and practical method. Chest *60*:73, 1971.

Furman S, Escher DJW: Temporary transvenous pacing, *in* Principles and Techniques of Cardiac Pacing. New York, Harper & Row, 1970.

Hindman MC, Wagner GS, Jaro M, et al: The clinical significance of bundle branch block complicating acute myocardial infarction. 1. Clinical characteristics, hospital mortality, and one-year follow-up. 2. Indications for temporary and premanent pacemaker insertion. Circulation *58*:689, 1978.

Lown B, Kosowsky BD: Artificial cardiac pacemakers. N Engl J Med *283*:907, 1970.

Meister SG, Banka VS, Helfant RH: Transfemoral pacing with balloon-tipped catheters. JAMA *225*:712, 1973.

Preston TA: A new temporary pacing catheter with improved sensing and safety characteristics. Am Heart J *88*:289, 1974.

Resnekov L, Lipp H: Pacemaking and acute myocardial infarction. Prog Cardiovasc Dis *14*:475, 1972.

Schnitzler RN, Caracta AR, Damato AN: "Floating" catheter for temporary transvenous pacing. Am J Cardiol *31*:351, 1973.

Solomon N, Escher DJW: A rapid method for insertion of the pacemaker catheter electrode. Am Heart J *66*:717, 1963.

14

INTRAAORTIC BALLOON COUNTERPULSATION

General Considerations

Definition: Intraaortic balloon counterpulsation (IABC) is a mechanical technique for reducing the left ventricular workload and also improving myocardial oxygen supply. A variety of intraaortic balloon pumps (IABP) are commercially available. The IABP is usually placed from the femoral artery (either by cutdown or percutaneously) with the balloon located in the descending thoracic aorta just distal to the left subclavian artery.

Instrumentation required:

Catheter with 30 or 40 cc balloon for adult IABC

Connecting tubing to allow the console to rhythmically inflate and deflate the balloon, using helium or CO_2

An intraarterial cannula (for timing of inflation/deflation with the arterial pulse wave) is frequently placed in a radial or brachial artery. A recent innovation allows the aortic pressure to be monitored from the balloon tip.

Console (the display and controls, fault alarms, and pumping mechanism). The patient's ECG and the arterial pulse wave are used to time the inflation/deflation cycle for optimal counterpulsation.

Physiology of IABC

Diastolic augmentation: Displacement of blood by balloon inflation during diastole raises aortic diastolic pressure, increasing coronary blood flow and thereby myocardial oxygen supply. Balloon inflation is timed to occur at the closure of the aortic valve, as indicated by the arterial pressure dicrotic notch.

Systolic afterload reduction: Rapid balloon deflation during systole results in a small decrease in arterial systolic pressure (a decrease in afterload) and improvement in forward left ventricular stroke volume, by facilitation of ventricular emptying.

Timing of inflation/deflation: Because of the delay in arterial wave transmission to the radial artery and the delay in balloon inflation pressure wave from console to catheter tip, optimal inflation/deflation must precede the timing point just noted by approximately 50 msec. Optimal timing requires small adjustments of inflation/deflation until peak diastolic augmentation and systolic unloading are observed on the arterial pressure tracing.

Clinical Indications for Use of IABC

Acute Myocardial Infarction Shock

(also see Chapter 20)

Prerequisites for IABP use:

Early intervention, usually < 6 hours after the onset of symptoms of MI or extension

Instrumentation to assure that hypovolemia is not causally related (mean pulmonary capillary wedge > 18 mm Hg)

Depression of cardiac output (< 2.2 L/min/M^2)

Hypotension may not be present, although most patients having other prerequisites will usually have a systolic arterial pressure < 90 mm Hg.

Inability to normalize the above values with inotropic agents or afterload-reducing agents (when severe hypotension is absent) within 1–2 hours.

Results

Variable; this depends on the interval from onset of symptoms to institution of IABC, and the character of the patient group

Approximately 50–75% will achieve improvement of circulatory hemodynamics; 15% of those achieving hemodynamic stabilization can have the balloon gradually discontinued ("weaning"); 60–85% remain IABP-dependent and require surgical therapy for their survival. Approximately 50% of those without large aneurysms, extensive ventricular akinesis, or prior infarction damage will survive surgery. Survival is expected to be lower in patients with these additional factors.

Acute Mitral Regurgitation or Ventricular Septal Defect (VSD) During Myocardial Infarction

(also see Chapter 21)

Prerequisites

Pulmonary congestion as a result of mitral regurgitation or the left-to-right shunt of VSD

Diagnosis confirmed by Swan-Ganz catheterization (large V wave in wedged tracing [mitral regurgitation, MR] or ≥ 5% increase in oxygen saturation between right atrium and right ventricle [VSD])

A trial of afterload reduction (with nitroprusside) has been first undertaken without reduction of mean pulmonary capillary wedge pressure of V wave (MR), or mean PA pressure (VSD), and an improvement in respiratory symptoms. The effect is usually dramatic. A trial of 30–60 minutes is usually sufficient.

In the hypotensive patient (systolic blood pressure, < 90 mm Hg), afterload reduction generally should not be attempted; direct application of IABC is indicated.

Results

Most patients with a massive VSD or MR in the setting of acute MI suffer a very high mortality rate despite all medical and surgical measures.

If stabilization with IABC can be achieved and IABP discontinued, operation should be deferred to a time when the operative risk is reduced; at 3–6 weeks post-MI, it is reported that operative mortality is in the range of 15%; at 3 months, it is 5–10%. Those severely ill patients who respond poorly to afterload reduction and/or IABP therapy, and require surgery in less than 3 weeks, have a mortality rate of more than 30–50%.

Unstable Angina (also see Chapters 17 and 23)

Indications

For unstable angina unresponsive or poorly responsive to medical therapy. Patients with recurrence of angina more than 24 hours after an acute MI who are poorly responsive to drug therapy are also included in this group. The recent use of intravenous nitroglycerin and calcium-blocking agents such as nifedipine or diltiazem, in addition to standard beta-blockers and nitroglycerin, appears to be reducing this need for IABC. Early coronary angiography in the patient who is subsequently well controlled on medical therapy is frequently necessary.

Results

95-100% of patients can be expected to experience a reduction in the frequency of anginal episodes, with more than 75% having complete cessation of symptoms.

Cardiac catheterization and coronary arteriography are best performed soon after stabilization of symptoms. The IABP is usually left in place and functioning, which allows the catheterization procedure to be carried out without undue recurrence of symptoms.

Those with post-MI angina who stabilize on IABC are usually best weaned from IABC and allowed to undergo a period of recovery.

Long-term results in unstable angina depend on the coronary anatomy and ventricular function and are similar to those achieved when patients are stabilized on drug therapy alone.

Contraindications

Compromise of lower extremity circulation

History of intermittent claudication

Poorly palpable femoral pulses

Absence of popliteal or pedal pulses

Other signs of distal circulatory insufficiency (loss of hair, cold feet, poor capillary filling)

Aortic disease

Abdominal or thoracic aneurysm

Marked calcification and tortuosity

Disorders of clotting

Platelet count < 100,000

Coagulation factor deficiencies

Technique for Insertion and Removal

Cutdown Technique

Surgically placed in femoral artery

Prosthetic side-arm graft sutured to artery. Balloon and catheter passed through graft and femoral artery and positioned in aorta; entry site closed by tie around graft/catheter.

Removal under surgical conditions, with tie closure of the graft. If there are signs of distal arterial circulation compromise, Fogarty balloon removal of clots should be undertaken. Femoral cutdown site is then closed.

Percutaneous Technique

This is a new technique that allows IABC to be undertaken by the cardiologist or angiographer, with results comparable to those of the cutdown technique

Entry is from the femoral artery. The limb must have signs of good circulation, with readily palpable femoral arteries and present distal pulses.

By Seldinger technique, a 12 French (Fr) cannula is introduced into the femoral artery. Recent modifications include a longer cannula that can be advanced into the abdominal aorta and a balloon/catheter that itself can be advanced over a spring guidewire. Both modifications are intended to reduce the possibility of aortic dissection and facilitate passage of the intraaortic balloon.

The balloon is twisted on itself, passed through the catheter, and positioned at a predetermined length of catheter with its tip below the left subclavian artery. The cannula is left in place; a tie or special clamp is placed securely around the cannula and its contained catheter. Continuous drip heparin in therapeutic doses is given to prevent clots from forming on the balloon and catheter.

Placement is best achieved under fluoroscopic control. In all cases a postplacement chest radiograph should be obtained to assure and document position.

Removal. The femoral artery below the insertion site is completely obstructed by digital pressure, with proximal pressure toward the entry site. Following removal of the balloon the artery is allowed to bleed briefly, expression of any clots dislodged from the catheter during removal is accomplished by "milking" the artery proximally toward the balloon entry site.

Monitor distal pulses and circulation to detect compromise by embolization. Surgical removal of such emboli may be necessary.

Complications

Arterial dissection, 4%
Peripheral embolization requiring surgical removal, 10%
Sepsis of graft, incision, catheter/balloon
Platelet depression

REFERENCES

Gold HK, Leinbach RC, Buckley MJ, et al: Refractory angina pectoris: Follow-up after intraaortic balloon pumping and surgery. Circulation *54*(Suppl 3):41, 1976.

Resnekov L: Mechanical assistance for the failing ventricle. Mod Concepts Cardiovasc Dis *43*:81, 1974.

Scheidt S, Wilner G, Mueller H, et al: Intraaortic balloon counterpulsation in cardiogenic shocks: Report of a cooperative clinical trial. N Engl J Med *288*:979, 1973.

Subramanian VA, Goldstein JE, Sos TA, et al: Preliminary clinical experience with percutaneous intraaortic balloon pumping. Circulation *62*(Suppl 1):123, 1980.

Willerson JT, Curry GC, Watson JT, et al: Intraaortic balloon counterpulsation in patients with cardiogenic shock, medically refractory left ventricular failure and/or recurrent ventricular tachycardia. Am J Med *58*:183, 1975

IV

CCU TREATMENT OF MYOCARDIAL INFARCTION, ANGINA PECTORIS, AND THEIR COMPLICATIONS

15

ARRHYTHMIAS IN ACUTE MYOCARDIAL INFARCTION: RECOGNITION AND MANAGEMENT

CLASSIFICATION OF ARRHYTHMIAS

Supraventricular Versus Ventricular

Characteristics of ventricular ectopic beats or rhythms:

No associated P wave or atrial activity.

QRS widened (>90 msec).

Fully compensatory pause.

R on T and fusion beats may occur.

Ventricular rhythms may have dissociated atrial activity. Chance arrival of an atrial depolarization wave during a time when the AV node is not refractory may result in more normal ventricular conduction and thus a more normal QRS appearance (Dressler beat).

In V1, R higher than R′.

QS or rS in V6.

QRS all positive or all negative in V1–V6.

Characteristics of supraventricular ectopic beats or rhythms:

Abnormal P wave or other atrial activity may be associated but, because of a short coupling interval or rapid rate, may be hidden in the preceding T wave. For beats arising in the AV junction, atrial activity is frequently coincident with the premature QRS and therefore not seen.

QRS normal and similar to QRS of the regular rhythm *OR* may differ in configuration and width (minor aberration) *OR* may be abnormal in duration and configuration (major aberration). In the latter case, the QRS may resemble a ventricular ectopic beat.

Less than compensatory pause.

R on T unlikely (conduction through AV node unlikely during this refractory period).

The initial beat of a run may be recognized as a supraventricular beat.

In V1, R′ higher than R.

Triphasic pattern in V1 (rsR′) and V6 (QRS).

Initial QRS vector similar to normal beats.

More likely to occur following a normal beat that occurs after a pause.

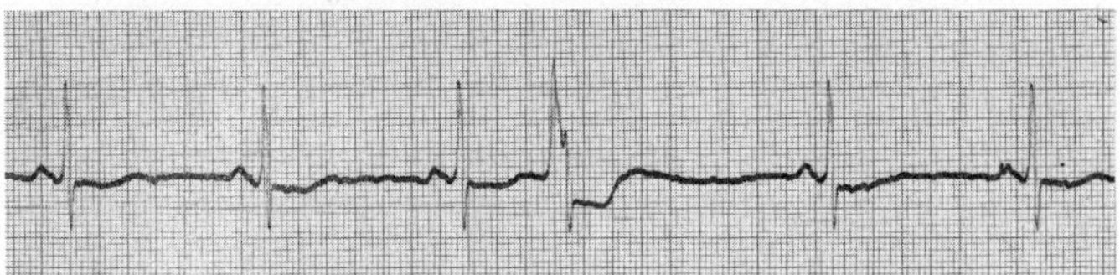

Figure 15–1. Sinus bradycardia with one ventricular premature beat.

Heart Block Rhythms

In the setting of conduction block, an escape rhythm will be seen; the rate and QRS configuration will depend upon the site of its origin. Dissociation of atrial and ventricular complexes occurs, with the atrial rate greater than the ventricular rate (see discussion in Chapter 13 on pacing).

IDENTIFICATION AND TREATMENT OF ARRHYTHMIAS

Sinus Rhythms

Rhythm originates in the "normal" site in the right atrium. Therefore, P wave is normal in vectorial direction and relation to QRS.

Sinus Bradycardia (Fig. 15–1)
Characteristics. Rate is <60/min. Frequently accompanies myocardial infarction (MI), especially with involvement of the inferior wall.
Significance. Of importance only if associated with signs of reduced cardiac output or hypotension. If nonsymptomatic, most authorities would leave untreated, since myocardial oxygen demand is consequently reduced. Conversely, most authorities would treat, despite absence of symptoms, if rate is in mid to low 40s or less. Controversy still exists about concurrent ventricular premature beats (VPBs); if infrequent and of the "escape" variety (occurring outside the T wave), many physicians would leave both the bradycardia and VPBs untreated, although atropine may abolish such ectopic beats.
Treatment. Atropine, 0.5 mg IV. May be repeated once or twice if the sinus rate fails to increase sufficiently, but be sure to allow 3–5 minutes to elapse between doses to avoid overdose and resultant tachycardia (which will increase myocardial oxygen demand and may precipitate angina). Avoid an initial dose of less than 0.5 mg (which may cause additional slowing).

If no adequate increase in rate with 1.5 mg IV over 10 minutes and there are signs or symptoms of hypotension/hypoperfusion: immediately place a temporary transvenous ventricular pacemaker

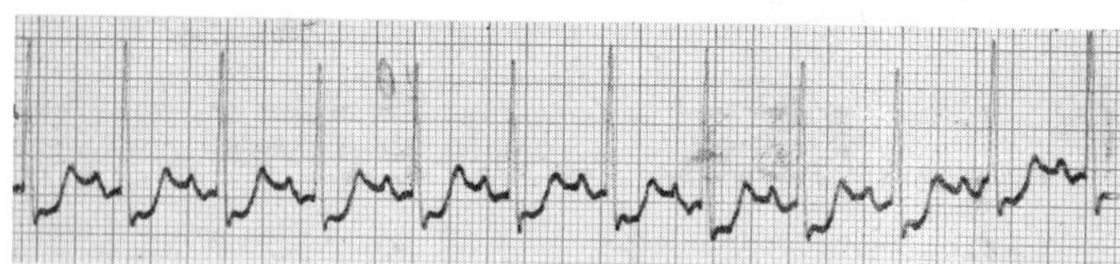

Figure 15–2. Sinus tachycardia in a patient with myocardial ischemia. Note ST segment depression.

(an atrial site may be advantageous if normal IV conduction is present). Avoid use of beta-stimulation (isoproterenol), which increases myocardial oxygen demand and may easily result in sinus tachycardia or ventricular ectopic arrhythmia (VEA) in the acute MI situation.

Sinus Tachycardia (Fig. 15–2)
Characteristics. Rate >100/min. Must be distinguished from supraventricular tachycardia, atrial fibrillation, or flutter. May show small variations in R-R interval; carotid massage may slow rate slightly and fails to reveal an underlying block.
Significance. Usually a response to the stress of the acute situation and should respond to rest and relief of pain and anxiety. Persistent sinus tachycardia may be due to reflex response to low cardiac output states, although fever, other pain, discomfort, or anxiety should be ruled out. Other manifestations of heart failure should be sought, and intracardiac instrumentation may be necessary for diagnosis.
Treatment. Usual treatment is of the underlying condition. If a low cardiac output state exists, it should be treated following the scheme outlined in Chapters 19 and 20. In the patient with acute MI, digitalis is rarely of benefit, although there is some indication that it may lower filling pressure without compromising output in the failing heart. The hyperadrenergic state syndrome (see Chapter 16) occasionally exists in the acute MI patient and is effectively treated with beta-blockade (propranolol). It should never be given without documentation of the absence of heart failure, preferably by measurement of intracardiac filling pressures and cardiac output.

Ectopic Supraventricular Arrhythmias

Atrial Premature Beats (APBs) (Figs. 15–3 and 15–4)
Characteristics. Premature beats with P wave and R-R interval that may differ from "normal." QRS aberration (with differences in QRS configuration or duration) occurs frequently.
Significance. Of little importance. May herald the development of supraventricular tachycardias (especially atrial fibrillation) or impending congestive heart failure. May also signal atrial infarction or ischemia.

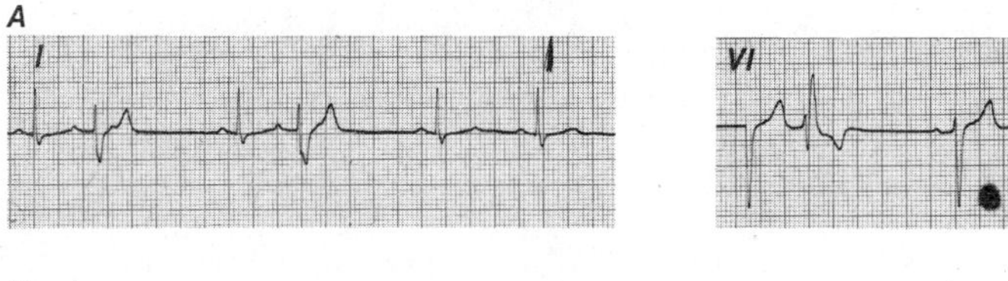

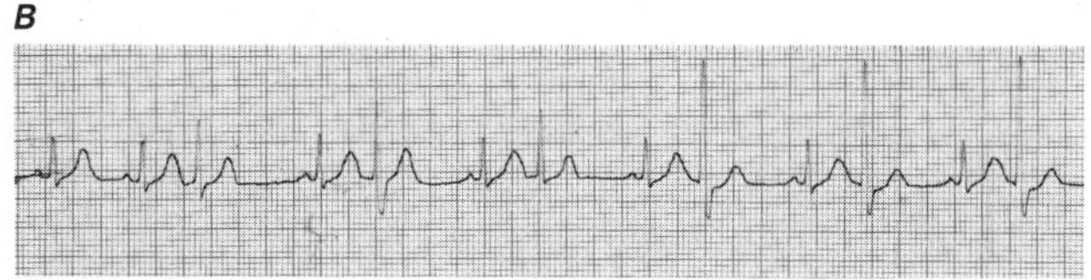

Figure 15–3. *A*, Atrial premature beats with aberration (wide QRS) are seen in Leads I and VI. *B*, Atrial premature beats showing a variety of aberrant ventricular forms, none of which is greater than 100 msec in duration.

Treatment. If infrequent, APBs require no treatment. Digitalization is usually beneficial if APBs are frequent, even in the absence of heart failure. Quinidine or procainamide may also be used.

Atrial Fibrillation (Fig. 15–5)

Characteristics. No organized atrial waves occur, and ventricular rhythm is regular. In most patients not receiving digitalis or beta-blockade, ventricular response is rapid (>140). Normal or slow ventricular rate in the absence of these agents should suggest an element of AV block.

Significance. The rapid ventricular rate is associated with increased myocardial oxygen demand and consequent increase in the extent of ischemia or infarction. There is also loss of atrial pumping function; if ventricular function is impaired, atrial fibrillation may result in a decrease in cardiac output, signs of impaired peripheral perfusion, or shock. With the higher ventricular rates, filling of the ventricle (a time-dependent phenomenon) is impaired and will result in a decrease in cardiac output. When a slow ventricular rate and ventricular ectopy are present, digitalis intoxication should be ruled out.

Treatment. With a *rapid* (>140/min) ventricular rate, *DC cardioversion* is the treatment of choice, especially in the setting of acute

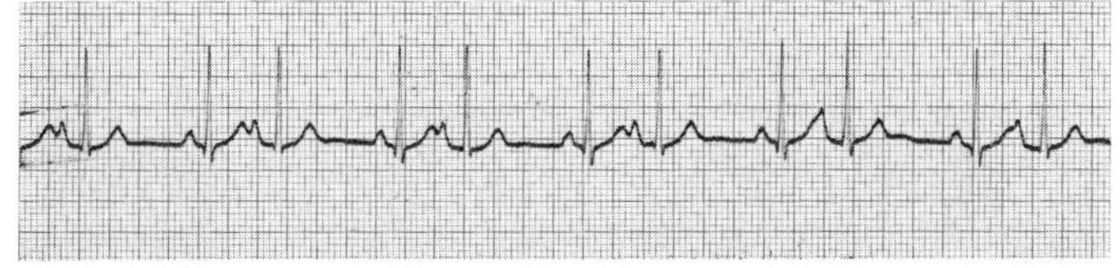

Figure 15–4. Atrial premature beats forming an atrial bigeminal rhythm.

A

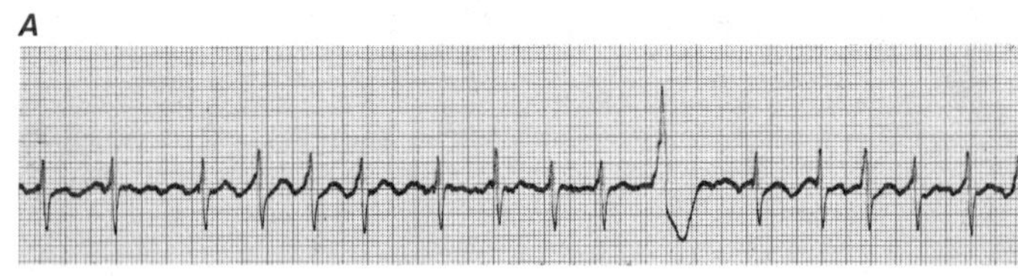

B

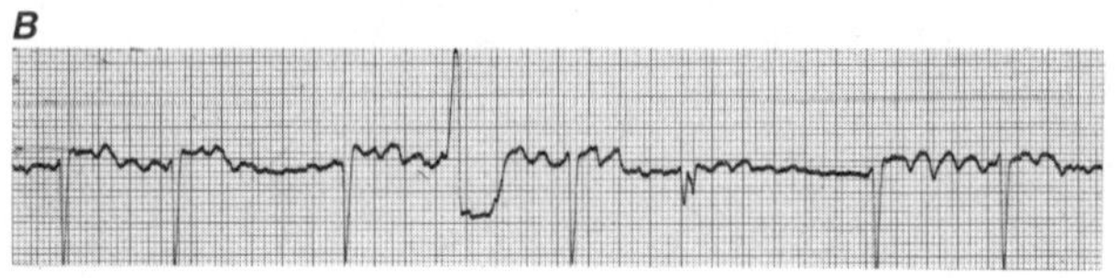

Figure 15–5. *A*, Atrial fibrillation with a rapid ventricular response (rate approximately 130). One ventricular ectopic beat. *B*, Atrial fibrillation with a slow ventricular response and ventricular ectopic beats. Digitalis excess should be considered.

infarction. For a *slower* ventricular rate, *rapid digitalization* should be instituted; digoxin, 0.5 mg initially (in divided doses if given IV), then 0.25 mg IV every 3–4 hours until the rate slows to <100/min or until 1.50 mg is given.

Extreme care must be exercised in the electrical conversion of patients taking digitalis, as therapeutic and high drug levels are associated with a high frequency of serious ventricular arrhythmias following countershock. It is wisest to avoid digitalis treatment in the patient in whom electrical conversion is considered a possibility and, of course, it is withheld if the rhythm suggests digitalis intoxication. Serum potassium should be measured and hypokalemia corrected if present.

Anticoagulation is not usually required for conversion of atrial fibrillation of short duration occurring in the acute MI patient.

Atrial Flutter (Fig. 15–6)

Characteristics. Rapid (280–350/min) atrial depolarizations are typically seen on the ECG as sawtooth waves. AV conduction block (2:1 to 4:1, or varying) occurs. Waves on occasion may be seen only in isolated leads, particularly V1 or V2. Changes in vagal tone, as a result of activity, vomiting, or vagomimetic drugs or during carotid sinus massage, will usually increase the block and more clearly demonstrate the atrial activity.

Significance. Usually seen in the presence of heart disease. As with atrial fibrillation, the resultant rapid ventricular rate may be detrimental to myocardial oxygenation and ventricular filling. Drugs, particularly quinidine, will result in a substantial increase in AV conduction and thus in ventricular rate. If given, such drugs must be administered concomitantly with digitalis to maintain AV conduction block.

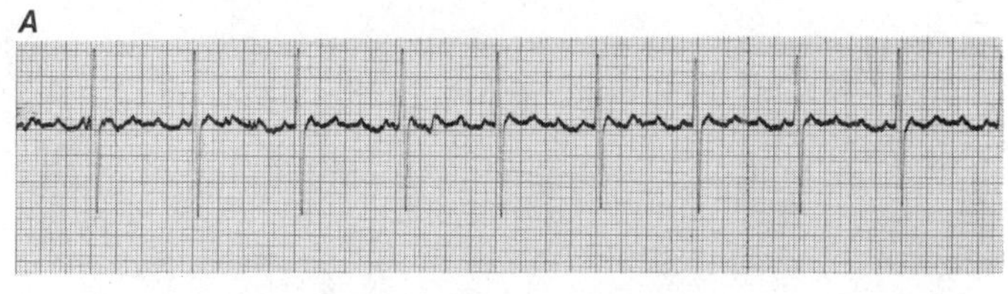

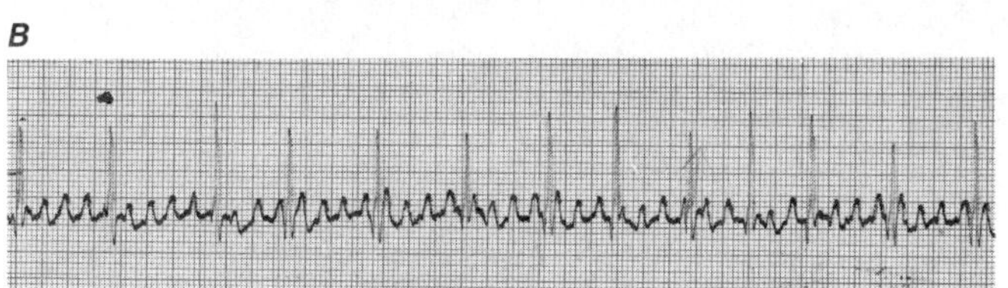

Figure 15–6. *A*, Atrial flutter (rate 300/min) with 4:1 block. *B*, Rapid atrial flutter (rate 260/min) with variable block.)

Treatment. In acute MI, the ventricular rate is usually difficult to control with digitalis, and attempts to do so usually result in the loss of valuable therapeutic time.

The *preferred treatment is electrical conversion,* which is often successful at low energy levels (25–50 joules) in returning the patient to sinus rhythm.

Paroxysmal Supraventricular Tachycardia (SVT) (Fig. 15–7)

This is a new designation for arrhythmias, previously known as paroxysmal atrial tachycardia (PAT) without block and junctional tachycardia, that have recently been shown to originate as reentrant rhythms from the AV node.

Characteristics. P waves may or may not be seen, depending on the relationship of atrial to ventricular depolarization.

Since these rhythms originate in the AV node, the rule is that no AV block is seen. (On rare occasions block may develop in the His-Purkinje system, making this arrhythmia appear similar to ectopic supraventricular arrhythmias with block.)

With vagal maneuvers (including carotid sinus massage), slight slowing occasionally occurs and the rhythm may abruptly terminate.

AV block does not occur nor is it induced by vagal maneuvers.

Significance. SVT is an infrequent occurrence in the patient with acute MI. It is usually a poorly tolerated arrhythmia; block does not occur and ventricular rates are usually fast; atrial and ventricular contractions occur simultaneously or nearly so, and the effect of atrial contraction on ventricular filling is lost.

Treatment. Prompt treatment is essential. Carotid sinus massage should be performed at once, first on one side, then the other. Failure of conversion to sinus rhythms should be cause for prompt synchronized electrical conversion. Continued atrial ectopic activity should be treated with IV or oral quinidine or procainamide. It is

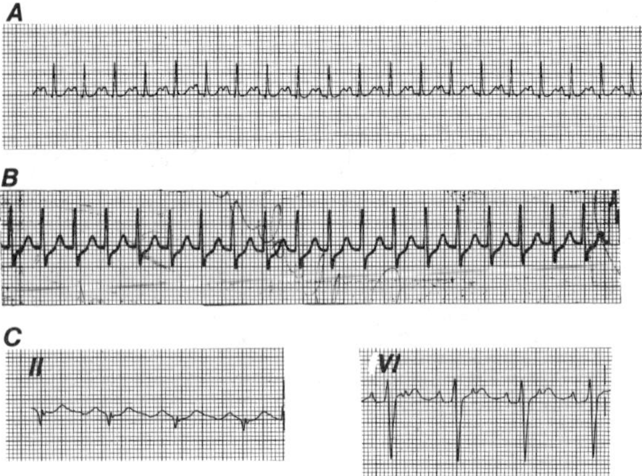

Figure 15–7. *A*, Supraventricular tachycardia (rate 200). P waves and 1:1 conduction can be easily seen. *B*, Supraventricular tachycardia (rate 190). No P waves are seen. *C*, Atrial ectopic tachycardia with 2:1 block in a patient with a recent inferior myocardial infarction. P waves are seen only in V-1. Digitalis toxicity was present clinically.

not appropriate to utilize pressors, Valsalva maneuver, or edrophonium (Tensilon) in the acute MI patient.

While verapamil is very effective in converting supraventricular arrhythmias, its use in the acute infarction patient should be limited to rhythms that are clearly supraventricular—that is, with normal QRS duration. Verapamil is given IV 5–10 mg over a 2 minute period; a second dose of 10 mg may be given in 30 minutes if initial conversion has not occurred, although DC cardioversion is the preferred treatment in this situation.

Ectopic Atrial Tachycardia

Characteristics. This is a new designation for arrhythmias previously known as atrial tachycardia with block; it includes some forms of atrial tachycardia without block as well.

Identifying signs include

P waves are different from the previous sinus wave.

There is usually an initial speeding up of the rate at initiation and then a stable atrial rate of 140–200/min, with AV block.

Since this is an arrhythmia originating from an automatic atrial focus, it is not initiated or terminated by ectopic activity or artificial pacing.

Vagal maneuvers may induce AV block but will not terminate the arrhythmia.

Significance. There is a high association of this rhythm with digitalis excess or intoxication. Since some patients with acute MI may be receiving concomitant digitalis, it is important to recognize drug toxicity as the major etiology. However, the acute MI itself may be responsible for this arrhythmia.

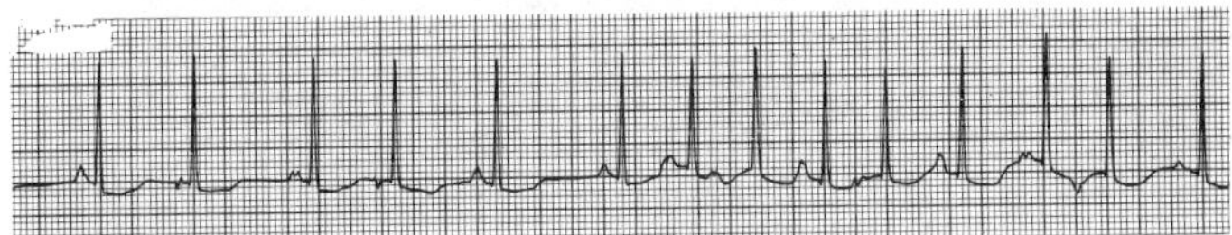

Figure 15–8. Multifocal atrial tachycardia with a markedly irregular ventricular rhythm that should not be confused with atrial fibrillation.

Treatment

If patient is receiving digitalis:

Hold further doses.

Check serum potassium. If low, correct with the addition of KCl supplements to the intravenous administration.

If urgent suppression of the arrhythmia is necessary, use of phenytoin (Dilantin) or propranolol to counteract the digitalis action may be effective.

Electrical reversion is contraindicated.

If patient is not receiving digitalis or digitalis intoxication is thought to be clinically unlikely:

Electrical reversion is considered to be the most efficacious treatment if hemodynamic compromise is present or the ventricular rate is high (>140; usually due to 1:1 conduction).

Otherwise, drug treatment is indicated. Digitalis will decrease atrial automaticity and decrease ventricular response to the atrial activity (induce AV block). Quinidine or procainamide will decrease atrial automaticity and both are also efficacious.

Other Supraventricular Reentrant Arrhythmias

SA Nodal Reentry. Normal P waves; AV block may exist; this is a recently described arrhythmia and is considered to occur infrequently.

Atrial Flutter. Actually a reentrant atrial mechanism; clinically considered individually and treated so here.

Multifocal Atrial Tachycardia (MAT) (Fig. 15–8)

Characteristics. Variable P-P′ and R-R′ intervals. P waves exhibit differing morphology in any given lead. Ventricular rhythm is irregular and rate varies (if APBs are frequent it may be high). May superficially resemble atrial fibrillation.

Significance. Usually found in the elderly or seriously ill and usually in association with chronic lung disease or metabolic disturbances (hypoxemia, hypokalemia). It must be distinguished from atrial fibrillation, since the usual therapy for atrial fibrillation is usually ineffective in MAT.

Treatment. Digitalis and other antiarrhythmic agents or electrical reversion is not effective. Treatment must be directed at the primary cause: hypoxia associated with chronic lung disease, congestive heart failure, electrolyte imbalance.

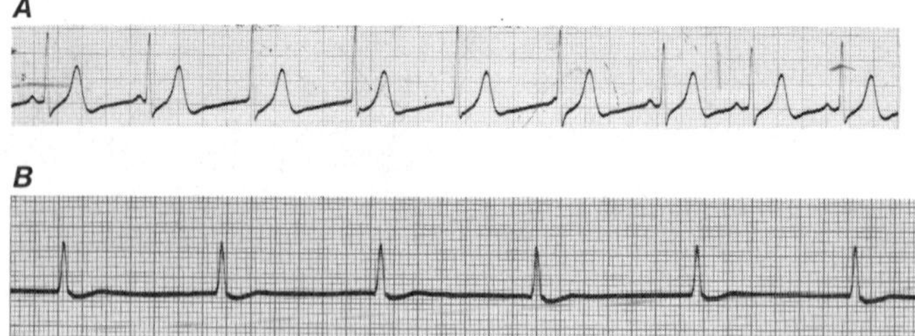

Figure 15–9. *A*, Normal sinus rhythm, usurped by an accelerated junctional focus. At the end of the strip, the sinus rate increases and assumes control. *B*, Junctional escape rhythm (rate 46/min) occurring in the absence of a faster atrial rhythm.

Accelerated Junctional Rhythm (Fig. 15–9)
Characteristics. Seen as a mild increase in junctional rate (60–90/min), which then exceeds the sinus rate, becoming a dominant rhythm. Since P wave and QRS are not related during periods when the junctional rhythm is dominant, this may be seen as a form of AV dissociation *without* AV block ("inteference dissociation").

In most cases it occurs during a phasic reduction in sinus rate and is consequently a transient phenomenon. Under these circumstances, when the two competing rhythms are at nearly identical rates, interference dissociation is referred to as "isorhythmic dissociation".

Ventricular conduction remains similar to that during sinus rhythm.

Should be distinguished from a junctional escape rhythm (rate <60), which may occur in complete heart block, and supraventricular tachycardia.

Significance. Occurs with a high degree of frequency in the acute MI setting. When transient, it is not usually associated with hemodynamic compromise.

Treatment. No treatment usually is indicated. Treatment is indicated when arrhythmia is continuous and accompanied by a fall in blood pressure or other signs of impairment in peripheral perfusion (due to loss of atrial function). Atropine is administered, using the sinus bradycardia protocol previously described to increase sinus rate. Atrial pacing can be used if atropine is ineffective, but this recourse is rarely needed.

Ventricular Arrhythmias

Ventricular Premature Beats (VPBs) (Fig. 15–10)
Characteristics. VPBs occur with a coupling interval less than the conducted rhythm. When the coupling interval approaches that of

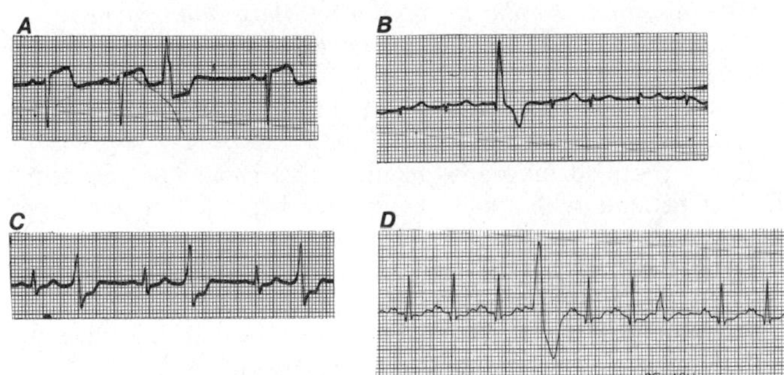

Figure 15–10. Ventricular premature beats *(A)*, with a prolonged coupling interval *(B)*, forming a bigeminal pattern *(C)*, and demonstrating multiform configuration with varying coupling intervals *(D)*. Note the short coupling interval in *D*. Compensatory pause is present in all four illustrations.

the conducted beat, a fusion beat occurs. Fusion is identified by configuration (containing elements between the VPB and normal QRS), variability (having slightly differing coupling intervals and QRS configuration changes), and usual association with nonfused VPBs.

Significance. In the patient with acute MI, VPBs may be associated with ventricular tachycardia or fibrillation.

Categories of VPBs considered harbingers (warning arrhythmias) of such life-threatening situations:

(1) VPBs with a frequency > 5/min

(2) VPBs occurring during the T wave of the preceding beat (the "R on T phenomenon")

(3) VPBs in pairs (couplets)

(4) VPBs of varying configuration (multiform)

(5) A "premature index" of less than 0.85 is considered by some authorities equally as important as the R on T. This is determined by dividing the interval of the VPB to preceding beat by the QT interval of the interval preceding the beat. The classification of R on T and low prematurity index as warning arrhythmias has recently been questioned. Most workers, however, continue to consider them so in the acute MI patient.

Treatment

Prophylaxis. Prophylactic use of lidocaine to prevent the emergence of VPBs and of ventricular fibrillation (VF) is recommended in all patients in whom acute MI is suspected, since more than 50% of VF episodes have no warning arrhythmia or occur too soon after the warning arrhythmia to be effectively prevented.

Contraindications

(1) The presence of second or third degree heart block

(2) Previous allergic reaction to lidocaine or related drugs

Administration (similar for both prophylaxis and treatment)

The use of a controlled infusion device is recommended to avoid lidocaine toxicity.

Doses are given IV over 1–2 minutes to avoid toxicity due to transiently high concentrations.

Doses (both loading and maintenance) should be reduced by half in patients with shock, congestive heart failure, or hepatic disease.

For the average sized patient, an IV loading dose of 75–100 mg is given, and an infusion of 3 mg/min started.

Additional doses of 50 mg each are repeated 2–3 times at 5 minute intervals (maximum loading dose is 225 mg).

For breakthrough ventricular arrhythmias, give 50 mg over 1–2 minutes and raise the infusion an additional mg/min. This can be repeated until infusion rates of 5 mg/min are achieved.

For breakthrough arrhythmia despite maximum lidocaine dose, discontinue maintenance lidocaine and give procainamide, 100 mg IV (slowly). Repeat every 5 minutes until arrhythmia is abolished or 1000 mg is given. Hypotension (from arteriolar dilation) occurs with rapid or excessive administration.

Suppression of VPBs after the Acute CCU Period

Procainamide, 250–500 mg orally every 4 hours. A sustained release form (Procan-SR) is now available and can be used if initial therapy is effective. Long-term treatment is associated with the appearance of antinuclear protein antibodies and lupus syndrome.

Quinidine may be used alternatively, although it has a high association with GI side effects: 300 mg orally every 6 hours.

Other Drugs. Beta-blocking agents or phenytoin can be tried for either acute or chronic treatment; they are rarely useful for treatment of ventricular arrhythmias. Disopyramide also may be used, although it is considered to be less efficacious and is associated with urinary retention and an increased incidence of heart failure.

Ventricular Tachycardia (VT) (Fig. 15–11)

Characteristics

Three or more VPBs in succession

Rate > 100/min, usually 140–200/min

Other characteristics of ventricular beats as previously outlined. Of particular help in differentiating VT from aberrantly conducted supraventricular rhythms is the presence of AV dissociation (with P waves at a slower rate) and Dressler beats.

Small degrees of irregularity sometimes occur at the beginning or end of a run.

Significance. Sustained VT is usually associated with hypotension and signs and symptoms of impaired peripheral perfusion.

In acute MI, sustained VT frequently degenerates into ventricular fibrillation.

Nonsustained VT frequently precedes more sustained VT and

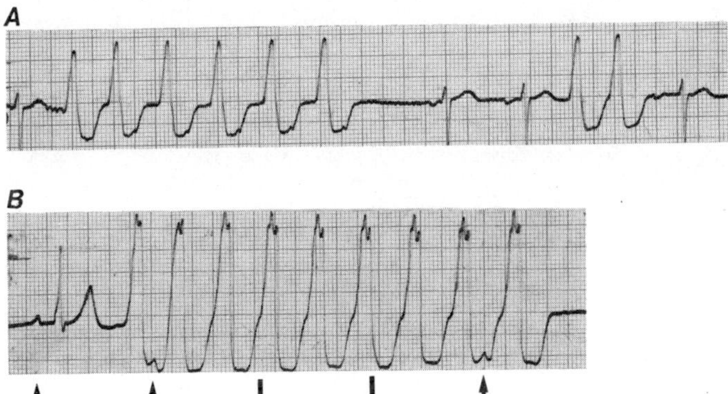

Figure 15–11. *A*, Nonsustained ventricular tachycardia (rate 120) demonstrating irregularity at the onset of the run. A ventricular couplet occurs later in the strip. *B*, Ventricular tachycardia (rate 135) showing independent P wave activity (arrows).

then VF. Brief runs may not be associated with abnormal signs or symptoms.

Treatment

Nonsustained VT

Immediately initiate lidocaine treatment. If patient is on lidocaine, increase dose as outlined earlier.

If ineffective, give procainamide as outlined earlier.

For recurrences of VT despite lidocaine or procainamide, a trial of bretylium is indicated:

—Give 5 mg/kg (300 mg for the average person) IV undiluted. If no response after 20 minutes, repeat a 10 mg/kg dose diluted in 50 ml of D5W or normal saline (NS) given over 10 minutes. Total dose should not exceed 30 mg/kg.

—Antiarrhythmic effects are usually delayed for 20–30 minutes, and initial response may be an increase in ventricular ectopic activity. Hypotension (particularly orthostatic) can be expected. Rapid injection is associated with nausea and vomiting.

—For maintenance, give 1–2 mg/min diluted in D5W or NS; 30 mg/kg/24 hr maximum dose.

Sustained VT

If the patient is on ECG monitoring, give a single precordial thump. This is not to be done in the unmonitored patient as it may result in ventricular fibrillation.

—*Conscious patient in absence of hypotension:* Lidocaine, 75 mg IV loading dose, and begin a drip of 3 mg/min. Additional 50 mg IV in 5 min. Prepare IV sedative and DC countershock.

—*Unconscious or conscious hypotensive patient.* Immediate synchronized DC countershock using 300 joules. It no reversion takes place, repeat immediately, using first 300, then 360 joules.

If ineffective, give procainamide, using protocol outlined under VPB treatment. Many authorities now recommend bretylium as a

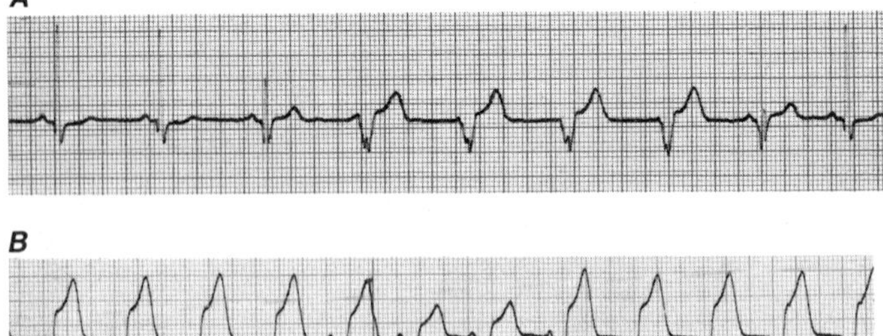

Figure 15–12. *A*, Accelerated idioventricular rhythm (rate 70) with initial and terminal fusion beats. *B*, Sustained AIVR (rate 97) with visible P waves and two capture beats (arrows).

"second-line" drug, using the protocol outlined under VPB treatment.

Repeated Episodes. Use the lowest energy level previously found effective; no additional benefit is accrued through the administration of higher levels.

Chronic Suppression (after the Acute CCU Period). Oral quinidine or procainamide, using the protocol outlined under VPB treatment.

Other Drugs. As with VPBs, beta-blockers, phenytoin, or disopyramide can be tried, but these are rarely effective.

Accelerated Idioventricular Rhythm (AIVR) (Fig. 15–12)

Characteristics

Runs of ventricular ectopic beats in series at a rate above sinus and <100/min

Characteristically consists of 3 or more beats but can be recognized as 2 when the condition is recurrent

Usually begins during the slow phase of sinus rhythm, with a long coupling interval (as escape beat)

Termination usually occurs with emergence of the sinus rhythm

Significance

Occurs in approximately 30% of patients with acute MI

Considered a benign occurrence not requiring treatment, unless associated with bursts of rapid VT

May cause hypotension from loss of atrial function

Some cases have been found to develop into VT. The majority of these have been described as beginning with a premature beat or as having a gradual acceleration to rates >110.

Treatment

Since AIVR represents an accelerated escape rhythm, increase of sinus rate will usually prevent its emergence. AIVR carries little

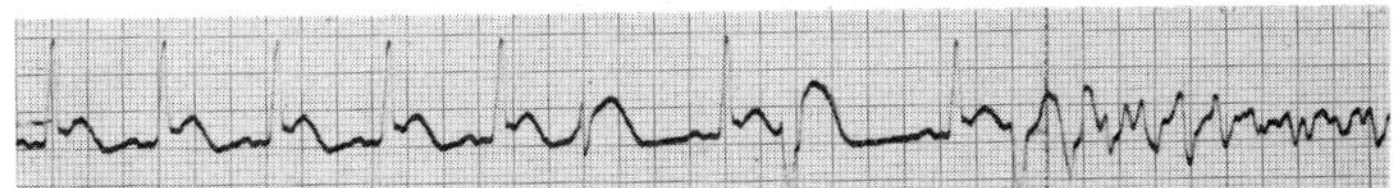

Figure 15–13. Ventricular fibrillation preceded by ventricular ectopic activity (note ST segment elevation).

risk, and there is usually little reason to attempt to override it (e.g., with atropine) or to suppress it (e.g., with lidocaine).

When hypotension occurs, give atropine IV, 0.5 mg repeated once or twice. In unusual situations, when there is failure of the sinus rate to increase sufficiently, an atrial pacemaker may be necessary.

Patients with acceleration in rates to levels > 110/min should be treated following the VT protocol.

Ventricular Fibrillation (VF) (Fig. 15–13)

Characteristics. Unorganized; rapid spike potential or varying amplitude and frequency. No recognizable complexes are seen.

Significance. Results in loss of all cardiac pumping function. Must be corrected as soon as possible. In a CCU, reversion within 30 seconds should be the norm. Success of resuscitative efforts declines markedly if VF continues untreated for more than 4 minutes.

Treatment. Immediate *unsynchronized* DC countershock using 300 joules. In the CCU patient not previously in shock, this can be expected to be 100% successful and should precede all other resuscitative measures.

Immediate IV lidocaine administration, using the protocol outlined under VPB treatment.

If DC reversion is not successful, repeat DC countershock immediately at 300 joules.

If unsuccessful, initiate Basic Life Support; repeat DC countershock, at 360 joules, after lidocaine loading and after correction of hypoxia, pH, and hypokalemia.

For recurrence despite maximal lidocaine treatment or for cases resistant to the measures just described, administer bretylium using the protocol outlined under VT treatment.

EMERGENCY SYNCHRONIZED DC CARDIOVERSION

Indications

(1) Tachyarrhythmias in which hemodynamic compromise is present

(2) Tachyarrhythmias in acute MI when the rate is fast (>140/min). Under these circumstances, increases in ischemia and infarct size are expected.

Contraindications

(1) Arrhythmias possibly due to digitalis excess

(2) Arrhythmias in patients receiving digitalis (a relative contraindication). Recent work suggests that few adverse effects occur in the absence of symptoms of digitalis toxicity.

(3) The patient with acute MI and atrial fibrillation in the setting of valvular disease or atrial dilation may not remain in sinus rhythm. However, synchronization remains indicated when hypotension or a rapid ventricular rate is present.

Procedure

Synchronization. The synchronizer should be turned on. The device will now seek a QRS of sufficient amplitude to activate that circuit. In the absence of such a QRS (such as during VF), the cardioverter will fail to fire.

QRS. The QRS should be upright, using a lead with maximal amplitude.

Energy level. Because of the seriousness of the situation, energy levels for emergency cardioversion are based on the necessity to effect immediate reversion. Other lower energy settings are usually indicated for elective cardioversion and are not discussed here.

Energy levels for the initial countershock remain controversial. Recommended levels are 50–200 joules. Atrial flutter usually will respond to the lower recommended level. In general, the 200 joule level should be used for all other situations.

Discharge. The buttons on both paddles must be depressed simultaneously and held during a brief pause while the device seeks a QRS complex.

If initially unsuccessful, repeat, using levels recommended for VF.

REFERENCES

Braunwald E (ed): Heart Disease: A Textbook of Cardiovascular Medicine. Philadelphia, WB Saunders Company, 1980, pp 630–743.

Chadda KD, Lichstein E, Gueta PK, Kourtesis P: Effects of atropine in patients with bradycardia complicating myocardial infarction. Am J Med *63*:503, 1977.

Engel TR, Meister SG, Frankl WS: The "R on T" phenomenon. Ann Intern Med *88*:221, 1978.

Epstein SE: Redwood DR, Smith ER: Atropine and acute myocardial infarction. Circulation *45*:1273, 1972.

Harrison DC: Should lidocaine be administered routinely to all patients after acute myocardial infarction? Am Heart J *58*:581, 1978.

Josephson ME, Kastor JA: Supraventricular tachycardia: Mechanisms and management. Ann Intern Med *87*:346, 1977.

Lichstein E, Ribas-Meneclier C, Gupta PK, Chadda KD: Incidence and description of accelerated ventricular rhythm complicating acute myocardial infarction. Am J Med *58*:192, 1975.

McIntyre KM, Lewis AJ (eds): Textbook of Advanced Cardiac Life Support. Dallas, TX, American Heart Association, 1981.

Shine KI, Kastor JA, and Yurchak PM: Multifocal atrial tachycardia: Clinical and electrocardiographic features in thirty-two cases. Circulation *36*(Suppl II):236, 1967.

Wyman MF, Lalka D, Hammersmith L, Cannom DS, Goldreyer BN: Multiple bolus technique for lidocaine administration during the first hours of an acute myocardial infarction. Am J Cardiol *41*:313, 1978.

16

MEDICAL MANAGEMENT OF ACUTE MYOCARDIAL INFARCTION

GENERAL CONSIDERATIONS

Next to the treatment of arrhythmias, the medical management of acute myocardial infarction is perhaps the single, most important task for the physician and nurse in the CCU. As discussed in detail in Chapter 2, myocardial infarction is a complex event still incompletely understood. Coronary occlusion produces myocardial necrosis, acute (often focal) left ventricular dysfunction, and a variety of arrhythmias. This "event" may not be a simple "all-or-none" phenomenon; indeed, the time-course of ischemic necrosis (infarction) of the left ventricle and the appearance of complications (most notably arrhythmias and heart failure) may vary widely from patient to patient. It is not surprising that universal agreement about the medical management of myocardial infarction is lacking, since our understanding of the pathogenesis of this complicated phenomenon is constantly evolving.

CLINICAL IMPLICATIONS

The approach to the patient with suspected acute myocardial infarction embodies four separate, but related, objectives that will be discussed individually.

Pain Relief, Sedation, Bedrest

The importance of relieving myocardial ischemic chest discomfort and allaying anxiety in the patient with acute myocardial infarction cannot be overemphasized. Often in this critical initial time period the relationship between physician and patient becomes firmly cemented.

In the very early phase of myocardial infarction, *autonomic imbalance* is frequent—either parasympathetic or sympathetic overactivity. In the former case, hypotension and bradycardia may supervene following inferior or posterior wall infarction. Such a preponderance of vagal-mediated manifestations (nausea, vomiting, bradycardia, and hypotension) may contribute to ischemic myocardial discomfort and may be exacerbated by the administration of certain narcotic agents—particularly morphine sulfate. In such instances, meperidine (Demerol) may be much more efficacious for analgesia and sedation, since its vagolytic effects are known to increase heart rate to more normal levels.

In contrast, some patients exhibit *sympathetic overactivity* in the early phase of acute myocardial infarction, characterized by tachycardia and mild hypertension. In such cases of this anxiety-induced "tachycardia-hypertension" syndrome, a loud first heart sound and wide pulse pressure may provide clinical clues to its presence. However, tachycardia may also represent the heart's response to severe left ventricular damage rather than simply sympathetic overactivity. The sympathetic overactivity syndrome can be treated by sedation, including morphine sulfate or meperidine: if symptoms persist, small doses of beta-blockers can be administered if the clinician can be certain that early left ventricular failure has been excluded. We feel that a pulmonary artery (PA) catheter is necessary to make this exclusion.

For *analgesia* in acute myocardial infarction or unstable angina, *morphine* continues to be the drug of choice. Meperidine (Demerol), hydromorphone (Dilaudid), and pentazocine (Talwin) also have been utilized but are much less effective in relieving the severe pain of acute myocardial infarction, except as just noted. Some investigators advocate the use of *nitrous oxide* (laughing gas) for the control of pain after acute myocardial infarction. This agent causes central nervous system sedation, relief of anxiety, and analgesia. It has negligible effects on heart rate and blood pressure, and left ventricular function appears to be not adversely affected by inhalation of a mixture of N_2O and oxygen. The use of nitrous oxide, however, involves a relatively complicated protocol for titration of optimal amounts of N_2O and O_2 and is generally reserved for patients who have persistent chest discomfort unresponsive to traditional nitrate and/or narcotic therapy.

As noted in Chapter 2, *ischemia* in a setting of coronary artery disease depends on changes in preload, afterload, contractility, and heart rate. Clearly, increases in these critical variables may often result in an imbalance in myocardial oxygen consumption relative to oxygen supply, such that increases in heart rate, contractility, or cardiac filling pressure may accelerate $M\dot{V}O_2$ and aggravate myocardial ischemia. Thus, it follows that therapy for ischemic chest discomfort should be ideally designed to decrease ischemia.

Increasingly, *nitroglycerin* (both sublingual and intravenous) has been used to relieve myocardial ischemia and chest pain. Several reports indicate that nitrate preparations used in patients who have normal-to-elevated left ventricular filling pressures may decrease electrocardiographic and enzymatic indices of acute myocardial injury. Although it is unclear whether these agents favorably influence myocardial infarct size, many cardiologists and internists advocate the use of sublingual or intravenous nitroglycerin as an initial analgesic agent in patients with acute myocardial infarction. However, since tachycardia and hypotension may be aggravated by the use of nitrates in patients with low cardiac filling pressures (decreased pulmonary capillary wedge pressure), invasive monitoring is often recommended if such continuing therapy is contemplated.

In addition to analgesics, *sedation* and *bedrest* are important in the very early phase of acute myocardial infarction. As a general rule, patients with uncomplicated infarction are allowed to use the commode during the first 24 hours in the CCU (see Chapters 6 and 7). Minor tranquilizers such as diazepam (Valium), chlordiazepoxide (Librium), and oxazepan (Serax) often promote suitable daytime sedation and alleviation of anxiety. This may be important also in the suppression of anxiety-induced arrhythmias.

Removal of Aggravating or Precipitating Factors in Myocardial Ischemia

As noted, the sympathetic and parasympathetic nervous systems have been found to play an increasingly important role in the genesis of myocardial ischemic chest pain. The presence of tachycardia, hypotension, and hypercontractility, as well as impaired myocardial contractility, may influence acutely the myocardial oxygen supply/demand ratio. Similarly, hypertension may accelerate the impedance to left ventricular outflow and augment myocardial oxygen requirements during ischemia. Congestive heart failure with elevated left ventricular filling pressure may increase oxygen requirements both by its effect on heart size and fiber length (preload) and wall tension (afterload). Clearly, the recognition of any of these conditions is critically important in the early management of patients with myocardial infarction, since the correction or treatment of these variables may favorably influence disproportionately elevated myocardial oxygen consumption.

Specific management of the aggravating or precipitating factors in myocardial ischemia will be discussed in detail in succeeding chapters.

Pharmacologic Reduction of the Determinants of Myocardial Oxygen Demand

Nitrates. Experimental and clinical studies have shown that acute myocardial infarction is a dynamic process unfolding over many hours. Reduction of oxygen consumption and/or work in the early phase of infarction may prevent necrosis and promote salvage of ischemic tissue. Conclusive evidence, however, is lacking that acute pharmacologic interventions can reduce infarct size (see also Chapter 24). The major effects of nitrates are to dilate venous capacitance vessels more than arteriolar resistance vessels, significantly reducing preload. Thus, in patients with acute infarction complicated by left ventricular failure, nitrates have been shown to decrease left ventricular end-diastolic and pulmonary capillary wedge pressures while maintaining cardiac index, heart rate, and stroke volume. Experimentally, nitrates are known to decrease coronary collateral flow resistance, increase collateral flow, and improve the endocardial/epicardial flow ratio in ischemic zones for sustained time periods.

Tachycardia and systemic arterial hypotension with decreased coronary artery perfusion, however, may occur during nitroglycerin administration in uncomplicated myocardial infarction (pulmonary capillary wedge pressure < 11 mm Hg). When systemic arterial pressure is low or borderline, or when there is suspicion that the left ventricular filling pressure may be normal or reduced, nitrates may pose a significant hazard.

The currently available nitrate preparations include traditional sublingual nitroglycerin, oral isosorbide dinitrate, sustained release oral nitroglycerin, nitroglycerin ointment, transdermal "patch" nitroglycerin, and intravenous nitroglycerin. In general, it is recommended that patients with presumptive myocardial infarction should receive initially 1 tablet (0.3 or 0.4 mg) of sublingual nitroglycerin for relief of ischemic chest discomfort. Careful monitoring of heart rate and blood pressure should accompany nitroglycerin administration. Should hypotension ensue, the patient should be placed in the Trendelenburg position, and IV fluids should be administered to replenish volume. If there has been a favorable therapeutic effect following the first nitroglycerin tablet and no untoward effects have developed, a second nitroglycerin tablet may be administered 15–20 minutes later.

Cutaneous nitrates are much longer acting than sublingual nitroglycerin, and their hemodynamic effects may persist for up to 3 hours after application. The transdermal patch form of administration has effects lasting a full 24 hours. In patients who have tolerated sublingual nitroglycerin without adverse effects, topical nitroglycerin may promote a more continuous preload reduction and relief of ischemia. Again, this form of therapy is much more efficacious in patients with left ventricular failure (see Chapter 19) and is considerably more hazardous in patients with low or normal left ventricular filling pressure. Since the dose response range is broad and variable, it is best to begin with 0.5 to 1 inch of nitroglycerin ointment every 6 hours or the lowest dose of the "patch" (5–10 mg). If this dose is tolerated without adverse hemodynamic effects, the regimen may be increased up to 2 inches every 3–4 hours as tolerated.

Intravenous nitroglycerin has been shown to be a valuable tool for the relief of ischemic chest discomfort in patients with myocardial infarction. At present, controversy persists about the efficacy of intravenous nitroglycerin in the setting of acute myocardial infarction, but several studies have reported the favorable effects of prolonged nitroglycerin infusion in these patients. The plasma half-life of nitroglycerin appears to be approximately 2 minutes in human beings because of redistribution and rapid hepatic metabolism. Accordingly, nitroglycerin can be used very effectively when acute nitrate therapy is necessary for preload reduction and/or relief of refractory myocardial ischemia. Because intravenous nitroglycerin may produce profound changes in left ventricular filling pressure, it is mandatory that this be used in a controlled setting where the patient can be invasively monitored on a continuous basis by skilled personnel in a CCU.

The preparation and use of intravenous nitroglycerin solution is discussed in detail in Chapter 19.

Propranolol. Because of its profound negative inotropic and chronotropic effects, the use of propranolol in acute myocardial infarction poses obvious hazards. Since myocardial necrosis produces segmental and global depression of left ventricular function, propranolol has generally been proscribed in the management of acute myocardial infarction. More recently, however, studies have been performed in patients with uncomplicated infarction to see whether the hemodynamic modification produced by propranolol could in effect reduce the area of myocardial injury.

While some investigators have reported initial success with combined intravenous and oral propranolol in patients with acute myocardial infarction, at present we are reluctant to treat patients with uncomplicated infarction with propranolol unless they exhibit persistent chest pain and ongoing ischemia associated with tachycardia *NOT* responsive to nitrates and analgesics. In our experience such patients are few, but we have found that if the pulmonary capillary wedge pressure is normal and tachycardia is not explained on the basis of pain or hypovolemia, the judicious administration of propranolol, 0.1 mg/kg IV, followed by oral propranolol in doses of 20–40 mg every 6 hours, has been effective for the relief of refractory pain.

We believe, however, that such treatment should be reserved only for those cases as detailed and should not be recommended as conventional therapy at this time.

Digitalis. Digitalis glycosides are effective for decreasing left ventricular filling pressure in patients with acute myocardial infarction complicated by congestive heart failure. However, digitalis administration remains controversial for patients with uncomplicated acute myocardial infarction, and it appears that its utility in such patients is negligible.

Other Antianginal Therapies. A new class of antianginal medication is available for the treatment of variant angina pectoris caused by coronary artery spasm and for angina pectoris that is medically refractory to conventional nitrate/beta-blocker therapy. These agents are known as calcium channel blockers, calcium antagonists, or calcium inhibitors. Their role in the setting of acute myocardial infarction remains undefined. They will be discussed in detail in Chapter 17.

Mechanical Reduction of Determinants of $M\dot{V}O_2$— Use of the Intraaortic Balloon Counterpulsation (IABC) Pump

The hemodynamic consequences of intraaortic balloon counterpulsation (IABC) are ideally suited for the preservation of ischemic myocardium, and IABC has been shown to be efficacious for this purpose experimentally. The intraaortic balloon is effective in lowering the pressure in the aorta at the time of opening of the aortic valve, which facilitates emptying of the left ventricle and decreases left ventricular volume. This decrease in left ventricular volume and the lowering of the impedance pressure against which the ventricle contracts affect two major determinants of the wall tension in the ischemic left ventricle—that is, reduction in ventricular pressure and diameter. By lowering tension in the myocardial wall, oxygen consumption ($M\dot{V}O_2$) is diminished and, thus, marginally ischemic myocardium may be preserved as oxygen requirements and oxygen supply are brought back into balance.

The use of IABC within the early hours of the onset of infarction has markedly improved many patients with hyperacute infarction who are experiencing persistent ischemic chest pain with evidence for accelerating electrocardiographic injury (ST segment elevation) and who are otherwise refractory to medical therapy. We have observed several such patients with markedly elevated ST segments whose signs of electrocardiographic injury were acutely reduced as the IAB was activated.

A recent report (Leinbach et al) of 11 patients with acute evolving anterior wall myocardial infarction less than 6 hours old revealed that half the patients experienced a rapid drop in ST segments with preservation of precordial R waves, following the insertion of the IAB within 2 hours of the onset of their myocardial infarction. The remaining patients who were classified as poor responders evolved electrocardiographic Q waves across the precordium despite a 40% drop in ST segment elevation with the institution of IABC. Subsequent coronary arteriography in all patients disclosed that all of the good responders had some residual patency of the left anterior descending coronary artery, while all but one of the poor responders had total occlusion of this vessel. Thus it does appear that IABC is efficacious in certain individuals who are refractory to conventional medical therapy but that at present it cannot be advocated for routine use.

We believe that if patients exhibit intensifying myocardial ischemia or electrocardiographic injury in the face of persistent ischemic chest pain not relieved by opiates or intensive nitrate therapy, prompt intraaortic balloon counterpulsation for the relief of ischemia and the salvage of ischemic myocardium is indicated. Clearly, this should be undertaken only by an experienced team in a properly monitored CCU setting, and in a patient in whom salvage of life or a significant amount of potentially viable myocardium appears reasonably likely.

The intraaortic balloon is discussed also in Chapters 14, 20, and 21.

REFERENCES

Armstrong PW, Walker DC, Burton JR, et al: Vasodilator therapy in acute myocardial infarction: A comparison of sodium nitroprusside and nitroglycerin. Circulation *52*:1118, 1975.

Corday E, Corday SR: Advances in clinical management of acute myocardial infarction in the past 25 years. J Am Coll Cardiol *1*:126, 1983.

Crexells C, Chatterjee K, Forrester JS, et al: Optimal level of filling pressure in the left side of the heart in acute myocardial infarction. N Engl J Med *289*:1263, 1973.

Forrester JS, Diamond G, Chatterjee K, et al: Medical therapy of acute myocardial infarction by application of hemodynamic subsets. N Engl J Med *295*:1356; 1404, 1976.

Gunnar RM, Loeb HS, Scanlon PJ, et al: Management of acute myocardial infarction and accelerating angina. Prog Cardiovasc Dis *22*:1, 1979.

Leinbach RC, Gold HK, Harper RW, et al: Early intra-aortic balloon pumping for anterior myocardial infarction without shock. Circulation *58*:204, 1978.

Mueller HS, Ayres SM: Metabolic responses of the heart in acute myocardial infarction in man. Am J Cardiol *42*:363, 1978.

Willerson JT, Buja LM: Cause and course of acute myocardial infarction. Am J Med *69*:903, 1980.

17

MEDICAL TREATMENT OF UNSTABLE ANGINA AND PRINZMETAL VARIANT ANGINA

UNSTABLE ANGINA

Unstable angina, or acute coronary insufficiency, has gained widespread acceptance during the last decade as a distinct clinical entity within the clinical spectrum of ischemic heart disease, bridging the gap between chronic stable angina and acute myocardial infarction. The definition of unstable angina pectoris remains controversial and has been plagued by a plethora of terms that have been used interchangeably over the course of the last decade to emphasize the critical nature of this syndrome. Thus, the terms unstable angina, acute coronary insufficiency, preinfarction angina, crescendo angina, and intermediary coronary syndrome have all been used synonymously in describing this syndrome.

In general, a suitable definition of unstable angina should embrace one or another of the following historical features:

(1) classic Heberden's angina of new onset, that is, usually within 1 month;

(2) development of crescendo (more severe) pain superimposed on a preexisting stable pattern of effort angina; or

(3) development of angina at rest.

Within the broad context of this definition, episodes of pain may be discrete as well as multiple, and there may be overlap among the three features just listed. Clearly, the characteristics of the chest pain in this syndrome are similar to those of classic, effort-induced angina, although the pain or discomfort is usually more prolonged and intense. Often, it may appear at rest and may frequently wake the patient from sleep ("nocturnal angina"). Unlike chronic, stable angina pectoris, which typically is promptly responsive to sublingual nitrates, unstable angina is usually protracted in nature, of at least 20 to 30 minutes' duration, and with incomplete or no relief following nitrate administration.

PRINZMETAL (VARIANT) ANGINA

A special category of patients with unstable angina includes those with the clinical presentation of cyclic, recurrent chest pain at rest that is unrelated to effort but is associated with ST segment elevation on the resting ECG. Patients with this variant form of angina (Prinzmetal angina) frequently describe prolonged attacks of chest pain, which sometimes occur at the same time each day, often in the early morning. Since its initial description by Prinzmetal in 1959, the incidence of this syndrome is still unknown.

The ECG demonstrates striking ST segment elevation with reciprocal depression during an attack, which subsides completely as these self-limited episodes of rest pain abate. Arrhythmias, particularly ventricular, are known to occur more frequently than in other anginal syndromes, being present in almost half these patients. Frequently, patients are thought to be evolving an acute myocardial infarction; however, administration of nitroglycerin promptly relieves the pain and ST segment elevation in most cases. Recent studies have shown conclusively that dynamic coronary obstruction is responsible for the chest pain and transmural electrocardiographic injury in this subset of patients. although a large proportion of individuals exhibit underlying fixed coronary stenosis as well.

Thus, it is becoming increasingly clear that unstable angina and Prinzmetal variant angina may share a common pathophysiologic basis, and both entities may represent an aborted myocardial infarction. It is felt that many patients with unstable angina and Prinzmetal variant angina experience a dramatic reduction in myocardial oxygen supply, although it is uncertain whether high-grade fixed coronary obstruction alone or critical coronary luminal narrowing with *superimposed* spasm is the responsible pathogenetic mechanism. The hypothesis that transient coronary spasm may be responsible for these multiple ischemic episodes that often herald acute myocardial infarction has obvious therapeutic implications, which will be discussed in detail.

RECOMMENDATIONS FOR TREATMENT OF UNSTABLE ANGINA AND PRINZMETAL ANGINA

A clinican confronted with a patient presenting unstable angina must decide on the best treatment for that particular individual. In general, either drug therapy or mechanical assistance with intraaortic balloon counterpulsation can be employed.

Drug Therapy

Nitrates. The utility of nitrates and beta-blockers in patients with unstable angina in the absence of acute myocardial infarction is well documented. Hesitancy in using nitrates in patients in whom myocardial infarction is suspected has been predicated on the agent's potential for causing excessive hypotension and thus reducing coronary arterial perfusion. Nitrates can be given sublingually or cutaneously; however, in unstable angina there may be certain advantages in using a continuous nitroglycerin infusion, since the dose can be carefully adjusted to achieve the desired effect while at the same time avoiding hypotension and/or reflex tachycardia. Additionally, the relief of angina during IV nitroglycerin administration has recently been reported in patients who previously failed to respond to sublingual administration. Thus, we recommended the use of sublingual nitroglycerin on a prn basis for unstable angina and the institution of long-acting nitrate therapy (nitroglycerin ointment 2%, in a dose ranging from 1–2 inches q 4 hr as tolerated). We prefer to use intravenous nitroglycerin in patients with evidence of unremitting angina and/or electrocardiographic evidence of intensifying ischemia who have not responded to intensive cutaneous nitrate therapy.

Obviously, hypotension and tachycardia are known side effects of intensive nitrate therapy, and individuals must be monitored closely to observe for these side effects. The question thus arises as to whether it is necessary to monitor left ventricular filling pressure routinely in all patients, using a Swan-Ganz catheter, before giving intravenous nitrates or beta-blocking agents. We prefer this approach only in the hypotensive patient. Our initial recommendation is to use intravenous nitroglycerin in prepackaged sterile ampules (Nitrobid, Tridil). Each vial contains 10 ml of a 50 mg solution of sterile intravenous nitroglycerin, diluted in 500 ml of dextrose and water. The initial infusion rate ranges from 5–10 μg/min, although we have employed doses safely in excess of 200 μg/min. The infusion is discontinued if (1) systolic blood pressure falls below 100 mm Hg; (2) a greater than 20 mm Hg decline in systolic blood pressure occurs; and (3) heart rate increases beyond 110 beats/min. In general, since intravenous nitroglycerin exerts its major effect on the coronary conduit and venous capacitance vessels and not the arteriolar resistance vessels, hypotension and reflex tachycardia are generally not observed within the recommended dosage range.

Beta-Blockers. Beta-blockers, of course, may further depress an already impaired left ventricle, and it has been suggested that use of these agents in clinical situations when coronary spasm is highly suspected (Prinzmetal variant angina) may produce unopposed alpha-adrenergic tone (facilitated vasoconstriction), thereby exacerbating vasospasm. However, studies have long supported the favorable effect of combination nitrate/beta-blocker therapy because of the well-documented decrease in myocardial oxygen demand and the increase in myocardial oxygen supply. Thus we believe that most patients with unstable angina should be given beta-blockers. The majority of these individuals will respond to intensive oral therapy; patients with intensifying ischemia or refractory angina or both may require intravenous propranolol. Small amounts of propranolol (1 mg) IV are given, repeating the dose every few minutes until a maximum of 0.1 mg/kg of body weight has been achieved as a loading dose over approximately 20–30 minutes. This should be followed immediately by oral propranolol, since the half-life of intravenous propranolol is short. We generally commence therapy with 40–80 mg po q 6 hr as tolerated.

The patient will have a Swan-Ganz catheter inserted only if he or she appears to be having hemodynamic difficulty or if there is a question of whether propranolol is inducing cardiac failure. If propranolol induces bradycardia at relatively low dose ranges, a pacemaker catheter can be inserted for the purpose of maintaining heart rate at a safe level while propranolol therapy is continued. Every effort should be made to interrupt this syndrome of accelerating angina, and analgesics, including opiates, will be used as needed. In addition, the patient should receive nasal oxygen, heparin by constant IV administration or by bolus infusion, and strict bedrest.

Calcium Channel Blockers. The role of coronary artery spasm in the pathogenesis of various myocardial ischemic syndromes, such as unstable angina—and certainly Prinzmetal's variant angina—has received considerable attention during recent years. Some patients with unstable angina, either pre- or postinfarction, show classic ST segment elevation during pain, a finding highly suggestive of coronary spasm. In the great majority of patients with hemodynamic measurements made before and during their ischemic episodes, ischemia appears to develop prior to any increase in myocardial oxygen demands, suggesting a sudden reduction of regional myocardial blood flow as the cause. This is of particular importance since, in addition to nitrate therapy, the calcium channel blocking agents, particularly nifedipine and diltiazem, appear to be highly efficacious in terminating and preventing myocardial ischemia induced by coronary spasm.

Calcium ions play a very important role in the cardiovascular system. They are involved in electrophysiologic processes, link excitation to muscular contraction, control energy storage and utilization, and constrict vascular smooth muscle in coronary and systemic arteries. Although structurally dissimilar, all these calcium channel blocking agents inhibit the passage of calcium ions across cell membranes during the slow inward current of cellular depolarization, "uncouple" excitation-contraction, and dilate vascular smooth muscle.

These calcium channel blocking agents have multiple hemodynamic effects that make them potentially valuable in treating many cardiovascular disorders. The individual calcium channel blockers have different relative potencies on various cardiovascular functions. The net hemodynamic and electrophysiologic effect of each agent, therefore, results from a complex interplay of direct and reflex phenomena. The clinical efficacy of these agents in classic angina pectoris relates to their ability to decrease afterload, myocardial contractility, and heart rate and increase coronary blood flow.

Three calcium channel blocking agents are approved for use in this country: nifedipine (Procardia), verapamil (Isoptin, Calan),

Table 17–1. RELATIVE CARDIOVASCULAR EFFECTS IN VIVO

	NIFEDIPINE	VERAPAMIL	DILTIAZEM
Vascular Smooth Muscle			
Systemic vascular resistancc (SVR)	↓↓↓↓	↓↓↓	↓↓
Coronary vascular resitance (CVR)	↓↓↓↓	↓↓	↓↓↓↓
Electrophysiologic			
Heart rate	↑↑↑	0/↓ Ex	↓
PR interval prolongation	0	↑↑	↑↑
Ventricular			
Cardiac output	↑↑	↑/↓	↑
LVEDP	↑	0/↓	↓
– inotropy	↑/↓	↓↓	0
$M\dot{V}o_2$	↓	↓↓	↓

LVEDP, left ventricular end-diastolic pressure; $M\dot{O}_2$, myocardial oxygen consumption; Ex, exercise

and diltiazem (Cardizem). The agents that have been used most successfully to prevent coronary spasm in Prinzmetal's variant angina and in unstable angina are nifedipine and diltiazem (Table 17–1). Both are potent dilators of coronary arteries, although it appears that nifedipine has a proportionately greater effect on peripheral arterial vessels, which may induce a reflex-mediated adrenergic activity. This effect is not seen with diltiazem, which appears to exert a preferential vasodilatory effect on the coronary vascular bed.

The usual dose of nifedipine is 10–40 mg po q 6 h, and this regimen has proved very effective in the great majority of patients with vasospastic angina (Table 17–2). The dosage of diltiazem ranges from 120–360 mg/24 hr in divided doses. Diltiazem seems to be ideally suited for the management of patients with unstable angina or Prinzmetal variant angina because of its preferential

Table 17–2. COMPARATIVE PHARMACOKINETICS

	NIFEDIPINE	VERAPAMIL	DILTIAZEM
Dose	10–40 mg q 6–8 hr	80–160 mg q 6–8 hr	30–90 mg q 6–8 hr
Onset of action	20 min (oral)	30 min	15 min
	2–3 min (SL)	—	—
Peak effect	1–2 hr	4–5 hr	30 min
Half life	4–6 hr	6–8 hr	4–6 hr
Excretion			
Renal (%)	~80	~70	~35
Fecal (%)	15	15	65

effect on the coronary arteries. In addition, diltiazem has the *least* negative inotropic effects of the available calcium channel blockers, thus making it especially useful in patients with depressed left ventricular function.

Verapamil, which has profound electrophysiologic effects on the slow inward current, is emerging as a valuable antiarrhythmic agent. Reentrant supraventricular arrhythmias, such as paroxysmal supraventricular tachycardia, are particularly amenable to treatment with intravenous verapamil. However, the negative inotropic effects of verapamil, and its proportionately smaller effect on the coronary and peripheral vascular beds, limit its usefulness as an agent for treatment of coronary spasm. The usual oral dose of verapamil is 80–120 mg po q 6–8 hr.

All these agents have been employed in combination with propranolol as an adjunct in the management of patients with chronic, stable angina pectoris, although the combined negative inotropic effects of verapamil and propranolol may pose hazards to patients with left ventricular dysfunction. The role of these agents, either alone or in combination with nitrates and beta-blockers, in the management of patients with unstable angina pectoris and myocardial ischemia needs to be determined prospectively.

Intraaortic Balloon Counterpulsation

The intraaortic balloon has been discussed in Chapter 14, and the pathophysiology of its usefulness will not be discussed here in detail. The success of intraaortic balloon counterpulsation can be attributed briefly to its unique hemodynamic effects—i.e., augmentation of diastolic arterial (coronary perfusion) pressure and the simultaneous systolic unloading of the left ventricle. It is clear that no single drug or drug combination can reproduce both these effects at the same time, since drugs that increase arterial diastolic pressure tend to increase myocardial wall tension and oxygen demand, while drugs that lower arterial diastolic pressure and left ventricular wall tension may reduce coronary blood flow.

Since intraaortic balloon counterpulsation is not without complications, we elect to reserve it for use in patients with unstable angina who appear to be at particularly high risk. Such patients include those who have unremitting angina refractory to drug therapy as previously outlined, patients with objective evidence for intensifying ischemia (episodic ST segment elevation or depression by ECG unresponsive to drug therapy), and patients with repetitive, drug-refractory, life-threatening arrhythmias in whom recurrent ischemia is suspected. In our experience, intraaortic balloon counterpulsation frequently may interrupt the malignant syndrome of unstable angina pectoris and may be effective in preventing myocardial infarction or in limiting infarct size.

Once the intraaortic balloon has been inserted and the patient stabilized, coronary arteriography is performed and coronary artery bypass graft (CABG) undertaken if feasible.

REFERENCES

Boden WE, Bough EW, Benham I, et al: Unstable angina with episodic ST segment elevation and minimal creatine kinase release culminating in extensive, recurrent infarction. J Am Coll Cardiol *2*:11, 1983.

Conti CR, Curry RC: Therapy of unstable angina, *in* Cohn PF (ed): Diagnosis and Therapy of Coronary Artery Disease. Boston, Little, Brown, 1979, p 333.

Co-operative Unstable Angina Study Group. Unstable angina pectoris: National Cooperative Study Group to compare surgical and medical therapy. II. In-hospital experience and inital follow-up results in patients with one, two and three vessel disease. Am J Cardiol *42*:839, 1978.

Gazes PC, Mobley EM, Faris HM Jr, et al: Pre-infarctional (unstable) angina—a prospective study—ten-year follow-up. Prognostic significance of electrocardiographic changes. Circulation *48*:331, 1973.

Maseri A, Severi S, DeNes M, et al: "Variant" angina: One aspect of a continuous spectrum of vasospastic myocardial ischemia. Am J Cardiol *42*:1019, 1978.

Pepine CJ, Conti CR: Calcium blockers in coronary heart disease. Mod Concepts Cardiovasc Dis *50*:61, 1981.

Prinzmetal M, Kennamer R, Merliss R, et al: Angina pectoris, I. A variant form of angina pectoris. Am J Med *27*:375, 1959.

18

HYPERTENSION COMPLICATING ACUTE MYOCARDIAL INFARCTION

General

Definition: Elevation of blood pressure during the early stages of acute myocardial infarction.

Although mean blood pressure is usually considered, it is easiest to categorize patients according to diastolic measurements, assuming a proportionate elevation of systolic pressure.

Categories:

Mild = diastolic 90–100 mm Hg

Moderate = 100–110 mm Hg

Severe ≥ 110 mm Hg

Presentation

History. Previous hypertension is frequently but not always present; patient may be using antihypertensive medication in a normally adequate dose.

Physical examination. Related to the basic process. For many patients without previous history, no physical findings may be present. Accurate blood pressure determinations are essential and require use of an appropriate-sized cuff.

Follow-up. The finding of an elevated blood pressure is reason for ordering appropriate repeat measurements:

Mild—in 15 minutes, then every hour until normal or until four serial measurements show no change

Moderate—in 15 minutes, then every 30 minutes until normal or until four serial measurements show no change

Severe—every 15 minutes until a decline is noted

Mechanism

Not well substantiated. Assumed to be related to sympathetic stimulation of peripheral arteries as a result of stress or anxiety; occurs more frequently in those with previously noted labile hypertension.

Therapy

Rest and sedation. This will be the treatment for the majority of patients, resulting in a decline of pressure to or near normal within 1–4 hours.

If decline of pressure is not seen within the first 1–2 hours in those with severe hypertension, additional measures should be promptly undertaken.

The case for additional therapy in those with moderate hypertension is not clear-cut and must be determined by the observed changes in blood pressure and the overall condition of the patient. In many patients, intravenous diuretics may result in a mild decrease of pressure.

Use of nitroglycerin as a peripheral vasodilator. Many cases of sustained moderate hypertension will respond to sublingual nitroglycerin or nitroglycerin paste with a gradual decline of arterial pressure. Patients with more marked elevations may respond but with a lesser magnitude of reduction. Care must be taken, however, to assure that sinus tachycardia or marked reduction of blood pressure does not occur; precautions should include the use of initially small doses of sublingual nitroglycerin (0.15 or 0.3 mg). The legs should be promptly elevated if pressure begins to fall rapidly or is accompanied by sinus tachycardia.

Afterload reducing agents. In moderate-to-severe, sustained hypertension, failure to achieve reduction with rest, sedation, or nitroglycerin preparations as just noted should be reason to institute blood pressure reduction by use of nitroprusside, in order to promote a reduction of excessive myocardial oxygen demand and its effect of increasing infarct size. While there have been experimental and clinical observations to suggest that nitroprusside may promote a "coronary steal" and infarct extension, this effect is overridden by its favorable effect of reducing oxygen consumption by the amelioration of hypertension in those with marked elevations of blood pressure.

The recommended initial dose of nitroprusside is 15 μg/min; the rate of infusion is increased every 3–5 minutes and the dose titrated to achieve normal systolic blood pressure (100–120 mm Hg). Effects are usually achieved at doses under 200 μg/min.

Thiocyanate is a normal metabolic product of nitroprusside and may be responsible for toxic symptoms: fatigue, anorexia, muscle spasms, and mental confusion or disorientation. The thiocyanate level should be followed if nitroprusside is administered for more than 48 hours, and the dose should be reduced or the drug discontinued if levels rise to more than 10 mg/dl.

Beta-blockade. Hypertension due to the sympathetic overactivity syndrome can be effectively treated by beta-blockade. However, caution must be taken to assure that this is not a reflex response to myocardial failure; when doubt exists, a Swan-Ganz catheterization should be undertaken to measure cardiac output and left ventricular filling pressure.

Sustained mild hypertension is best not treated acutely. Diuretics or other therapy can be utilized after 8–12 hours for gentle and long-term therapy. Some patients with moderate or severe hypertension may require chronic therapy; this decision should await 24–48 hours of the therapy just outlined.

REFERENCES

Chatterjee K, Parmley WW: Vasodilation therapy for acute myocardial infarction and chronic congestive heart failure. J Am Coll Cardiol *1*:133, 1983.

Chiariello M, Gold HK, Leinbach RC, et al: Comparison between the effects of nitroprusside and nitroglycerin on ischemic injury during acute myocardial infarction. Circulation *54*:766, 1976.

Shell WE, Sobel BE: Protection of jeopardized ischemic myocardium by reduction of ventricular afterload. N Engl J Med *291*:481, 1974.

19

LEFT VENTRICULAR FAILURE COMPLICATING MYOCARDIAL INFARCTION

GENERAL BACKGROUND

Left ventricular failure occurs as a consequence of insufficient cardiac output required to maintain adequate forward stroke output of the left ventricle at a level that satisfies perfusion of vital organs and tissues. In heart failure resulting from intrinsic myocardial damage, it is important to clarify how the ejection fraction and end-diastolic volume are affected. A direct consequence of myocardial damage is a reduced ability of the muscle fibers to contract, resulting in a decrease in the ejection fraction. Initially, this may be compensated for by ventricular dilatation, for, as the heart fails to eject an adequate stroke volume, diastolic volume increases, resulting in diastolic distention of the ventricle. Left ventricular end-diastolic pressure (LVEDP) rises as left atrial and pulmonary venous pressures rise. Such distention, by stretching the remaining intact myocardial fibers, may improve the performance of the heart by the Starling mechanism. However, ventricular dilatation is costly in other terms, for the dilated ventricle has a greater wall tension and consumes more oxygen than does a small ventricle. This poses limitations on the utility of ventricular dilatation as a compensatory mechanism, particularly when oxygen supply is limited as it is in ischemic heart disease.

LVEDP is quite commonly elevated in the acute phase of myocardial infarction. An elevated LVEDP, however, does not necessarily imply overt clinical left ventricular failure—that is, left ventricular S3 gallop and pulmonary rales. The pathogenesis for the rise in LVEDP in acute myocardial infarction (MI) relates to (a) left ventricular failure with a compensatory increase in left ventricular end-diastolic volume and pressure (Starling's law); or (b) decreased left ventricular compliance (increased stiffness of the left ventricular wall) and impaired ventricular relaxation. Commonly, an elevated LVEDP is the result of a combination of these two factors.

When the combination of new and old infarction compromises enough left ventricular mass, pulmonary venous congestion occurs as a manifestation of left ventricular failure. Hemodynamic evidence of systolic left ventricular dysfunction becomes apparent when 20–25% of the left ventricle is damaged; when 40–45% or more of the left ventricle is infarcted, power failure develops and cardiogenic shock ensues. These derangements in systolic function secondary to acute myocardial infarction often result in inadequate systemic perfusion with subsequent compensatory increases in left ventricular end-diastolic pressure and volume. Patients frequently exhibit cardiomegaly, pulmonary rales, and an S3 gallop.

If congestive heart failure is mild and not associated with progressive ischemia, this can be treated like other forms of congestive heart failure, with diuretics and digitalis. The particular features of acute myocardial infarction that make treatment unique, however, are the changes in diastolic compliance of the ischemic left ventricle that may contribute to an elevated LVEDP. Swan has demonstrated that during the phase of edema early in the course of myocardial infarction, when the ventricular wall is stiff, the ischemic myocardium presents an immobile baffle against which the remaining normal cardiac muscle can contract. This mandates that the remaining normal heart muscle must work at a higher filling pressure in order to move the ventricle to the optimal peak of the Frank-Starling curve. Even though this type of ventricle as a whole may be functioning in a "congestive failure" range with a high filling pressure and low cardiac output, it may respond very poorly to diuretics. Filling pressure and congestion are generally reduced but may result in a fall in cardiac output below levels necessary to sustain vital organ perfusion. Thus, this type of ventricle has need either for mechanical support or for the addition of an inotropic agent that will shift the Frank-Starling curve of the remaining normal myocardium up and to the left.

Frequently it is necessary to quantitate left ventricular filling pressure (pulmonary capillary wedge pressure) and cardiac output by invasive means with the use of a Swan-Ganz catheter, in order to plan most appropriately the proper therapy for patients with myocardial infarction (see Chapter 12). With a single catheter in the right side of the heart, the effects of acute myocardial infarction and its complications upon right atrial, pulmonary artery, and pulmonary capillary pressures, as well as cardiac output, can be assessed continuously. Alterations in the magnitude and morphology of intracardiac pressure wave forms are of major diagnostic importance in a number of pathologic cardiovascular conditions encountered in the Coronary Care Unit.

The most widespread application of hemodynamic monitoring of MI patients hospitalized in the CCU is the recognition of clinical and hemodynamic subsets based on the work of Forrester et al (see Chapters 11 and 20). Clinical subsets are defined by the manifestations of pulmonary congestion (reflecting increased pulmonary capillary pressure) and peripheral hypoperfusion (reflecting decreased cardiac output). On the basis of these findings, four clinical subsets are defined:

C-I, no pulmonary congestion or peripheral hypoperfusion;

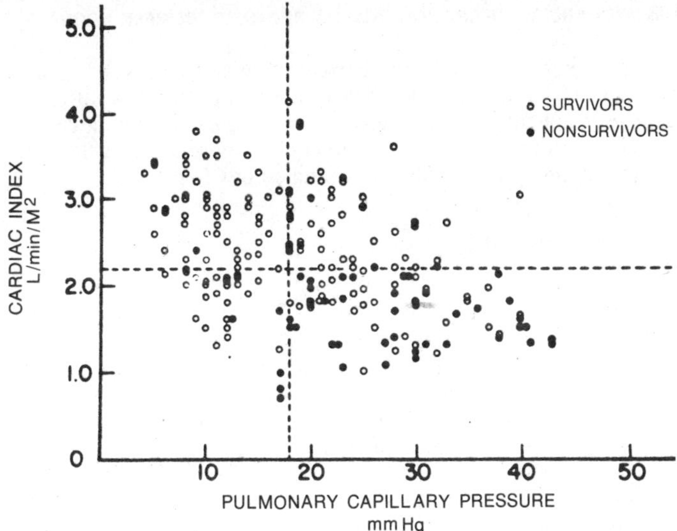

Figure 19–1. Relation between pulmonary capillary pressure and cardiac index in 200 patients at the time of admission to Cedars-Sinai Medical Center Myocardial Infarction Research Unit. The dotted lines are placed at the levels of 18 mm of Hg for pulmonary capillary pressure and 2.2 L/min/M^2 for cardiac index. A wide degree of variability in left ventricular performance in patients with acute MI is seen, and mortality rate increases as cardiac performance deteriorates.

(From Forrester JS, et al: Medical therapy of acute myocardial infarction by application of hemodynamic subsets. N Engl J Med *295*:1358, 1976.)

C-II, pulmonary congestion without hypoperfusion;
C-III, peripheral hypoperfusion without congestion; and
C-IV, both hypoperfusion and congestion.

These clinical subsets are of value in determining short-term prognosis. Although clinically uncomplicated MI patients virtually always survive hospitalization (1% mortality), the mortality rate increases to approximately 10% when pulmonary congestion is present and to approximately 60% when both pulmonary congestion and peripheral hypoperfusion are present.

Four comparable hemodynamic subsets are defined by the specific levels of cardiac index and pulmonary capillary wedge pressure. The comparable hemodynamic subsets are defined as follows (Fig. 19–1):

H-I, pulmonary capillary pressure $\leq$ 18 mm Hg and cardiac index > 2.2 L/min/M^2;

H-II, pulmonary capillary pressure > 18 mm Hg and cardiac index > 2.2 L/min/M^2;

H-III, pulmonary capillary pressure $\leq$ 18 mm Hg and cardiac index $\leq$ 2.2 L/min/M^2; and

H-IV, pulmonary capillary pressure > 18 mm Hg and cardiac index $\leq$ 2.2 L/min/M^2.

Clinical subset classification correctly predicts into which hemodynamic subset a patient will fall in approximately 70% of cases. As a result of this, the mortality rates in these four hemodynamic subsets are comparable to those in clinical subsets. (Specific treatment by hemodynamic subsets is detailed in Chapter 20).

RECOMMENDATIONS

Diuretics

Diuretic agents such as furosemide (Lasix) reduce pulmonary capillary pressure and cause little change in cardiac output or heart rate in patients with heart failure due to acute infarction. As noted, however, they must be used with caution in patients with myocardial infarction, since these individuals may require high filling pressure to sustain cardiac output. Lowering intracardiac filling pressure with a diuretic may well move the patient into a shocklike low cardiac output state. At present, the most common cause of hypovolemic shock in acute myocardial infarction is the overzealous administration of loop diuretics.

It has been shown that furosemide reduces pulmonary capillary pressure within minutes of administration and that these extrarenal effects on venous capacitance vessels precede the renal (diuretic) effects by approximately 15–30 minutes. Clearly, in patients with marked pulmonary congestion, the improved pulmonary compliance that occurs as the edema is cleared usually reduces the work of breathing, improves oxygenation, and markedly improves ventricular function by decreasing heart size and wall tension. However, these agents should be used cautiously in individuals who have borderline hypotension and probably should be used only if invasive monitoring is employed.

Digitalis Glycosides

Digitalis preparations are useful in the management of congestive heart failure complicating acute myocardial infarction. These agents have generally been proscribed because of the difficulty of detecting significant effect in the patient with uncomplicated acute myocardial infarction, and because of their capacity to produce arrhythmias when given in large amounts. Unquestionably, the digitalis glycosides improve left ventricular performance and contractility, particularly in patients with failing ventricles in whom the reduction in ventricular size decreases oxygen requirements more than the increase in contractility augments oxygen requirements. However, in the nonfailing, normal-sized left ventricle, there most likely is an increase in myocardial oxygen consumption that would vitiate any potentially beneficial increases in myocardial function.

It is emphasized that digitalis is a weak inotrope compared with sympathomimetic amines and, as such, does not precipitate inordinate rises in myocardial oxygen requirements as do the catecholamines. It has been shown that digitalis preparations do reduce end-diastolic pressure and volume as contractility increases. However, cardiac output may not increase.

As a general rule, digoxin is the agent of choice and it should be given in less than the full digitalizing dose to patients in congestive heart failure between 24 and 48 hours postinfarction. Thus, it is our practice to digitalize patients with evidence for large myocardial infarctions complicated by congestive heart failure with half the usual digitalizing dose during the first 48–72 hours of admission.

Vasodilators

In congestive heart failure, an increase in impedance to left ventricular ejection appears to be an important factor in impairing left ventricular performance. Arteriolar narrowing and decreased arterial compliance will decrease the left ventricular ejection fraction, while reduction in venous capacitance will shift blood centrally and increase cardiac filling. Vasodilator drugs, by relaxing the increased vascular tone, will reduce ventricular volume and increase stroke volume and thus improve the patient's hemodynamic and myocardial metabolic states.

Three agents most commonly employed are

(a) long-acting nitrates (cutaneous nitroglycerin ointment or isosorbide dinitrate),

(b) intravenous nitroglycerin, and

(c) sodium nitroprusside.

In patients with chest pain and acute MI, we commonly employ *sublingual nitroglycerin* and either *cutaneous nitrates* or *oral, long-acting nitrates.* Cutaneous nitrates especially are well absorbed, have a duration of action of 3.5 to 4 hours, and exert a significant decrease in left ventricular filling pressure and volume. However, for the management of patients with congestive heart failure secondary to acute myocardial infarction, we prefer to use parenteral agents, most notably intravenous nitroglycerin.

Nitroglycerin (Nitro-Bio, Tridil) is commercially available in sterile 10 ml vials containing 50 mg of nitroglycerin in solution. We dilute this in 500 ml of dextrose in water to obtain a concentration of 100 μg/ml. It is most appropriate to have an arterial monitoring line in the radial artery and a Swan-Ganz catheter in the pulmonary artery. Pulmonary wedge pressure can be checked periodically, but once the relationship between pulmonary wedge and pulmonary end-diastolic pressures is established, it is possible to follow the latter parameter as an index of left ventricular filling pressure.

While there may be a mild decrease in arterial pressure, intravenous nitroglycerin rarely causes hypotension or reflex tachycardia. By dilating larger *conductance* coronary arteries as well as smaller *collateral* vessels, intravenous nitroglycerin shifts blood flow toward the ischemic area, where arteriolar vasodilatation is preserved by the effects of ischemia. Clearly, its greatest physiologic effect is on the venous capacitance bed; with very little effect on systemic arteriolar resistance vessels, this agent is the parenteral vasodilator of choice in patients with left ventricular failure complicated by high pulmonary capillary wedge pressure.

Continuous infusion is initiated at 10 μg/min and increased 5–10 μg every 10 min. At doses above 80–100 μg/min, individual titration is required, and caution is advised. Generally, this dosage range is satisfactory for achieving the desired hemodynamic response (decline in left ventricular filling pressure) or clinical response (relief of angina, reversal of ischemic ECG changes) or both.

In the presence of systolic hypertension (> 170–180 mm Hg), *nitroprusside* may be the most appropriate vasodilator in the management of left ventricular failure, since this agent reduces both blood pressure and LVEDP. Its chief effect is on the arteriolar resistance vessels, but there is an effect on the venous capacitance vessels as well. It will increase the cardiac index in patients who have a low initial cardiac index and will decrease left ventricular filling pressure. This effect on improving cardiac index is in contrast to intravenous nitroglycerin, which has negligible effects on cardiac index and stroke volume. However, its use in acute myocardial infarction is still considered controversial, particularly in light of several experimental studies that have indicated that sodium nitroprusside may intensify ischemia by decreasing myocardial blood flow to ischemic left ventricular myocardium. In addition, clinical studies have indicated an increase in ST segment elevation in patients with acute anterior infarction. Although inconclusive, these data suggest the presence of a "coronary steal" syndrome, which may aggravate underlying myocardial ischemia and/or facilitate infarct extension.

Nitroprusside is available in 50 mg vials and is diluted in either 500 ml of D5W (100 μg/ml) or 250 ml of D5W (200 μg/ml). The solution may precipitate in a sodium chloride diluent and is extremely light-sensitive. Nitroprusside is generally begun at 10–15 μg/min and increased every 2–3 minutes until the pulmonary capillary wedge pressure falls to the 15–18 mm Hg range. Systolic arterial pressure should not be permitted to fall below 90 mm Hg since hypotension may aggravate coronary perfusion.

It is our view that nitroprusside should be reserved for the hypertensive MI patient characterized by an elevated peripheral resistance or systemic vascular resistance (SVR), or for the acute MI patient with congestive heart failure who has a depressed cardiac index and an elevated pulmonary capillary wedge pressure (Forrester subset IV) in whom IABP is not indicated. In normotensive MI patients with elevated left ventricular filling pressures unresponsive to loop diuretics, we prefer to utilize intravenous nitroglycerin alone or in combination with dobutamine (see Chapter 20).

Catecholamines

Norepinephrine (Levophed), dobutamine (Dobutrex), and dopamine (Intropin) are all utilized as adjuncts for the treatment of left ventricular failure complicating acute myocardial infarction. Dobutamine is currently regarded as the synthetic catecholamine of choice for patients with depressed cardiac output due to myocardial infarction. It has theoretic advantages over dopamine, since the latter tends to promote a greater heart rate response and may further elevate left ventricular filling pressure. These agents are discussed in detail in Chapter 20.

REFERENCES

Armstrong PW, Walker DC, Burton JR, et al: Vasodilator therapy in acute myocardial infarction. A comparison of sodium nitroprusside and nitroglycerin. Circulation *52*:1118, 1975.

Bussman WD, Passek D, Seidel W, et al: Prospective randomized trial of intravenous nitroglycerin in acute myocardial infarction. Circulation *59* (Suppl II):164, 1979.

Chatterjee K, Parmley WW: Therapy of acute myocardial infarction, *in* Cohn PF (ed): Diagnosis and Therapy of Coronary Artery Disease. Boston, Little, Brown, 1979, p 357.

Chatterjee K, Parmely WW: Vasodilator therapy for acute myocardial infarction and chronic congestive heart failure. J Am Coll Cardiol *1*:133, 1983.

Cohn JN: Vasodilator therapy of congestive heart failure. Ann Intern Med *26*:293, 1980.

Cohn JN, Franciosa JS, Francis GS, et al: Effect of short-term infusion of sodium nitroprusside on mortality rate in acute myocardial infarction complicated by left ventricular failure. Results of Veterans Administration Co-operative Study. N Engl J Med *306*:1129, 1982.

Durrer JD, Lie KI, Van Capelle FRJ, et al: Effect of sodium nitroprusside on mortality in acute myocardial infarction. N Engl J Med *306*:1121, 1982.

Forrester JS, Diamond G, Chatterjee K, et al: Medical therapy of acute myocardial infarction by application of hemodynamic subsets. Part I of two parts. N Engl J Med *295*:1356, 1976.

20

THE MYOCARDIAL INFARCTION SHOCK SYNDROME

General Considerations

Definition

The myocardial infarction shock syndrome is the acute inability of the heart to pump sufficient blood to meet demands of the body adequately. The term *myocardial infarction shock syndrome* has been used interchangeably with the more familiar *cardiogenic shock*. The former term is preferred, however, since cardiogenic shock implies that the myocardial damage is directly responsible for the shock state, while from a clinical point of view other factors (such as inadequate ventricular filling or myocardial suppression by extracardiac factors) may be responsible.

Etiology

It is generally accepted that most cases have infarction of at least 40% of the left ventricular myocardium. Acute myocarditis may occasionally present a similar clinical picture.

Presentation

Clinical Features

Restlessness; anxiety; peripheral vasoconstriction (cool, moist skin); impaired mental function; peripheral pulses usually faint and rapid; decreased urinary output (<20 ml/hr)

Hemodynamic Features

Cardiac index <2.2 L/min/M^2 BSA (body surface area)

In most situations, pulmonary capillary wedge (PCW) is more than 18 mm Hg but may vary depending on the state of hydration and operation of venodilator reflexes.

Hypotension. Formerly the "hallmark" of shock, now regarded as only one of its manifestations. Many patients with shock will have a systolic blood pressure of <90 mm Hg; previously hypertensive individuals in shock may have a systolic pressure above this (95–100 mm Hg, for example).

Therapeutic Maneuvers: Immediate

Pulmonary Edema (See also Chapter 19)

Rule out *respiratory insufficiency* (in which case morphine sulfate and oxygen by mask may be detrimental).

Administer *oxygen*. This should be by a method other than nasal cannula, which contributes very little to oxygenation in the acutely ill patient. In severely hypoxic patients, intubation and assisted ventilation may be necessary.

Morphine sulfate. Best given IV, 5 mg initially, then 2–4 mg after 10 minutes if no sign of improvement in the pulmonary edema is seen.

If improvement with these measures does not occur:

(1) An *IV diuretic* (furosemide) should be given. Initial dose is 40 mg. If a prompt effect on respiratory symptoms does not occur, the dose is doubled (80 mg); it may be doubled again to 160 and to 320 mg if ineffective. The mechanism of action is immediate dilation of the venous system; blood is shifted from the lungs to the periphery, with a resultant decrease in pulmonary capillary wedge pressure within 5 minutes of administration (reduction of preload). Diuresis occurs shortly thereafter, but the immediate improvement in clinical state is due to the extrarenal effect;

(2) As an alternative to or (in the case of severely resistant symptoms) in addition to preload reduction with an IV diuretic, *nitroglycerin* may be given. The mechanism of action is similar—venodilation with a resultant reduction of ventricular preload. Dose: 0.4 mg sublingual. Administer with care in the patient with low blood pressure and avoid it in those with a systolic blood pressure of less than 95 mm Hg. Hypotension due to nitroglycerin administration should be treated by elevation of the legs (Trendelenburg position).

Phlebotomy (100–500 ml) is indicated if these measures are not immediately effective in improving respiratory signs and symptoms.

Hypoperfusion (Presumed Low Cardiac Output)

Rule out obvious *hypovolemia* (history of excessive diuresis, prolonged pressor therapy, poor fluid intake). This suspicion should be accompanied by an immediate trial of fluid therapy following the guidelines below.

Pressor therapy. In the patient with severe coronary disease, a subnormal blood pressure causes a drop in coronary perfusion, with consequent increase in the area of infarction. Therefore, blood pressure should be maintained at the minimal acceptable level—90 mm Hg systolic. Norepinephrine (Levophed), 16–24 μg/min, or dopamine (5–10 μg/kg/min) should be initiated and titrated to maintain that level of blood pressure.

Diagnostic Approach

Alternate Etiologies

Consider (and rule out if possible):

Hypoxia or respiratory insufficiency

Sepsis

Pulmonary embolism

PULMONARY CAPILLARY WEDGE (mm Hg)

Cardiac Index (L/min/M²)	<18	>18
>2.2	SUBSET 1 Normal	SUBSET 2 Pulmonary Congestion
<2.2	SUBSET 3 Peripheral Hypoperfusion	SUBSET 4 Pulmonary Congestion Peripheral Hypoperfusion

Figure 20–1. (From Forrester JS, Waters DD: Hospital treatment of congestive heart failure; management according to hemodynamic profile. Am J Med *65*:173–180, 1978.)

Dissecting aortic aneurysm

Pericardial tamponade

Bradycardia. Should be suspected as a primary etiology only when marked—that is, below 40. It may contribute to the shock state at higher heart rates. It is recognized that increases in heart rate above 60 may improve perfusion, but a more detailed hemodynamic investigation is required. Therapy: atropine, 0.5 mg IV repeated once if insufficient response.

Ventricular or atrial tachyarrhythmias or heart block with slow ventricular rate

Vasodilator therapy, particularly intensive nitrate therapy

Hemodynamic Measurements

Immediate hemodynamic measurements are indicated. A flow sheet to record changes in vital signs, patient status, medications, and hemodynamic measures is essential to appropriate therapy.

Hypotension

If hypotension is the indication for consideration of the diagnosis of shock, repeated measurements of blood pressure by cuff should be made. If blood pressure is persistently below 90 mm Hg systolic or heart rate persistently greater than 110, instrumentation with an intra-arterial cannula is indicated.

Measure Pulmonary Pressures (See also Chapter 12)

Technique. Swan-Ganz type of floating catheter, inserted percutaneously via jugular or subclavian route. Brachial cutdown or percutaneous femoral techniques are also useful but less stable.

Measurements: Pulmonary capillary wedge, pulmonary artery systolic, diastolic, mean.

Interpretation (see Fig. 20–1—Forrester classification):

PCW <15–18 mm Hg: shock may be due totally or in part to hypovolemia.

PCW >18 mm Hg: left ventricular failure may be present. Decreased LV compliance, fluid overload, tamponade, or obstruction (i.e., mitral stenosis) is another possible cause.

Measure Intraarterial Pressure (See also Chapter 12)

Technique. Use intraarterial cannula inserted percutaneously for accurate determination of blood pressure. A central aortic position of monitoring line advanced from a brachial site of introduction is most accurate, but monitoring at the radial artery is usually satisfactory.

Measurements. Systolic, diastolic, mean.

Pressure may be as much as 50 mm Hg higher than that determined by cuff.

Measure Cardiac Output (See also Chapter 12)

Method. The thermodilution technique with the Swan-Ganz catheter is an easy and reproducible method for the determination of cardiac output (CO). It requires injection of a crystalloid solution through the catheter and a special bedside computer for the calculation. Iced (rather than room temperature) injectate is more accurate and is preferred. Rapid, smooth injection is essential to accurate and reproducible results. Hand injection is usually satisfactory, but an injection "gun" is available and gives better overall results. A change in injectate temperature must not occur between injection and the time of measurement. Therefore, hand contact of the injection syringe must be minimal. Some computers are able to measure automatically the injectate temperature as it traverses the catheter, avoiding this problem. Two or three determinations should be performed at each point of measurement and the results averaged. Determinations should usually be within 10% of the average. It one result differs from the rest by more than 20%, it should be discarded. If determinations vary considerably, additional measurements should be made. However, since 10 ml of injectate is usually required for each determination, frequent measurements of cardiac output will result in significant fluid administration. At times, readjustment of the tip of the catheter may correct the variation between individual measurements. The Fick or indocyanine green methods are also acceptable but are generally not easily performed in the CCU.

Nomogram for determination of body surface area from height and weight

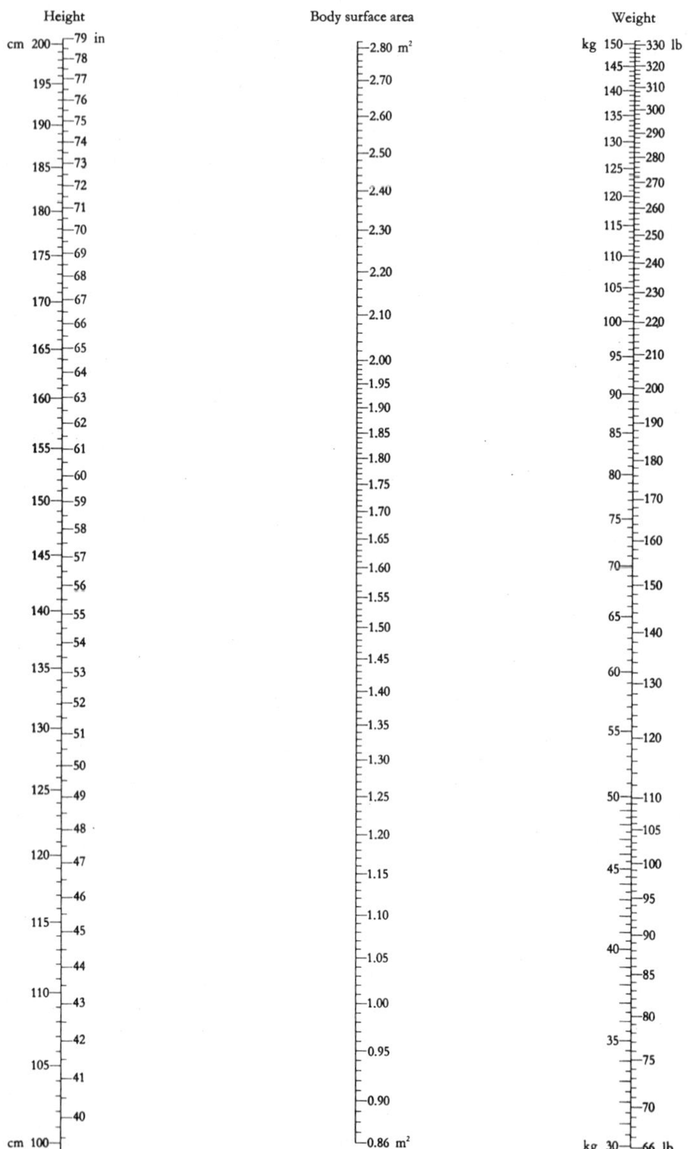

From the formula of Du Bois and Du Bois, *Arch. intern. Med.*, **17**, 863 (1916): $S = W^{0.425} \times H^{0.725} \times 71.84$, or $\log S = \log W \times 0.425 + \log H \times 0.725 + 1.8564$ (S = body surface in cm², W = weight in kg, H = height in cm)

Figure 20–2. Body surface area of adults. (From Geigy Scientific Tables. 7th ed. Ardsley, NY, Geigy Pharmaceuticals, 1970, p 537. Used with permission.)

Interpretation. Cardiac index (CI), to permit comparison among individuals of varying body masses, should be calculated. CI = CO ÷ body surface area (BSA). (See Fig. 20–2 for determination of BSA by body weight and height.) CI <2.2 L/min/M^2 of BSA is a major element of the definition of the shock syndrome. The thermally measured cardiac output is that of the *right ventricle* and may not reflect the totality of left ventricle output. This is of particular importance when elevation of right-sided pressure (e.g., due to RV infarction) causes right-to-left shunting through a patent foramen ovale.

Therapeutic Approach

Isolated Pulmonary Congestion (Forrester Subset II)

Findings

(1) Pulmonary capillary wedge >18 mm Hg

(2) Cardiac index >2.2 L/min/M^2 BSA

(3) Blood pressure normal (systolic > 90 mm Hg)

Treatment

(1) Diuretic agents. Reductions in cardiac output below an acceptable level by reduction of preload may occur. This will be evidenced by a drop in urine output, signs of decreased peripheral perfusion, or hypotension. In most situations, the left ventricle is operating on a depressed Frank-Starling curve, so that little change in cardiac output occurs, with modest reductions in preload.

(2) Intravenous nitroglycerin. This is a new modality available for the reduction of pulmonary congestion. While reductions of cardiac output due to a precipitous drop of preload are unlikely if the drug is administered in slow increments, a decrease in arterial pressure and increase in heart rate may occur at low dose, and frequent blood pressure measurements are essential. The recommended protocol is to begin with 5–10 μg/min and to increase the dose using the following schedule (μg/min): 10, 20, 30, 40, 60, 80, 100, 140, 180. Doses greater than 200 μg/min are infrequently needed.

Isolated Peripheral Hypoperfusion (Forrester Subset III)

Findings

(1) PCW < 15–18 mm Hg

(2) CI < 2.2 L/min/M^2 BSA

(3) BP usually low

Treatment

(1) This group of patients can be considered to be operating on a suboptimal portion of the ventricular function (Frank-Starling) curve. Increase in preload is frequently followed by increases in cardiac output, particularly if the PCW is < 12 mm Hg. The method of fluid administration must be cautious to avoid fluid overload and so that one can provide prompt information on the ability of the myocardium to respond with an improvement in

hemodynamics. Frequent small challenges are therefore recommended:

—A 100 ml bolus of fluid (normal saline or plasmanate) is injected over 1–2 minutes and the mean pulmonary capillary wedge observed.

—Additional boluses are given every 2–3 minutes until the PCW begins to rise. Then the interval between boluses is increased to 5 minutes.

—When the PCW is in the range of 15–18 mm Hg, cardiac output is repeated. In a few situations, the PCW may be raised above 18 mm Hg, but this should be done only if the situation is critical and then with great care, since pulmonary edema may be precipitated.

—Should the PCW rise abruptly above 18 mm Hg following a bolus, the challenge should be halted. In most cases the PCW will fall within a few minutes as the fluid becomes distributed.

—The decision about the type of injectate follows the nature of the response. In most cases, noncolloidal solutions are satisfactory and have the advantage of being excreted as cardiac function returns. A continued need for fluid administration, however, may require other materials that remain within the vascular system.

(2) In addition to the therapeutic nature of the fluid challenge, additional information about cardiac function is provided. Thus, individuals with isolated peripheral hypoperfusion who show little or no improvement in cardiac output despite increased PCW during challenge can be considered to have flat or poor ventricular function curves. The challenge therapy, by increasing the PCW, will then convert these patients into patients with combined pulmonary congestion and hypoperfusion (Forrester subset IV).

Complications. Pulmonary edema is the major adverse effect of treatment of this group. Should it occur, it should be treated promptly with IV diuretics, nitroglycerin, or phlebotomy.

Combined Pulmonary Congestion and Hypoperfusion (Forrester Subset IV)

Findings

(1) PCW > 15–18 mm Hg

(2) CI < 2.2 L/min/M^2 BSA

(3) Blood pressure < 90 systolic

Pharmacologic treatment to increase myocardial contractility

(1) Therapeutic maneuvers must be expediently undertaken since the mortality is high (60–80%); if these measures do not result in hemodynamic improvement over a 1–2 hour period, therapy should turn to mechanical support (provided the patient is a suitable candidate).

(2) Increase of myocardial contractility is the initial aim of therapy. Most clinicians and investigators favor dobutamine (250 mg/500 ml of diluent = 500 μg/ml) because of its positive inotropic

action with little direct systemic arterial constriction. Dosage: an initial 0.5 μg/kg/min. Usual range is 2.5–15 μg/kg/min.

Most patients at this stage will be receiving a pressor agent as part of the immediate therapy. This should be gradually decreased in dose as dobutamine is increased. Failure to maintain suitable blood pressure is an ominous sign, which requires that continuous pressor therapy be resumed.

Correction of hypoxia or acidosis may result in ability to reduce or discontinue pressors. The need for pressors otherwise represents an indication for mechanical support. Dopamine (200–400 mg/5 ml diluted in 250–500 ml of D5W or saline) may be used alternatively since it combines inotropic stimulation and renal vasodilation at a lower dosage (1–5 μg/kg/min). At moderate doses (6–10 μg/kg/min), peripheral vasoconstriction occurs and may reverse the renal effects as well as result in a primary increase in systemic blood pressure.

Other catecholamines that may be used include

—Norepinephrine (Levophed), which has primarily peripheral arterial (alpha) constrictor properties with some cardiac positive inotropic and chronotropic (beta) properties. The usual starting dose is 16–24 μg/min (1–2 ml/min of solution of a 4 mg vial in 250 ml D5W).

—Isoproterenol (Isuprel), which is a pure beta stimulant. Dilute 10 ml of solution 1:5000 (2 mg) in 500 ml of D5W. The usual starting dose is 2–20 μg/min, titrated to heart rate and onset of arrhythmias.

Neither norepinephrine nor isoproterenol are recommended because an increase in oxygen consumption and presumed increase in extent of infarction has been associated with their use. Norepinephrine, however, may be necessary to maintain blood pressure while instituting other measures.

—Vasodilators (also see Chapter 19)

—Diuretics (also see Chapter 19)

Complications of pharmacologic inotropic therapy

(1) Arrhythmias or sinus tachycardia, especially with isoproterenol or in dose ranges in excess of 20 μg/kg/min of dobutamine

(2) Increase in infarction size, as a direct result of myocardial stimulation and associated increase in myocardial oxygen demand

Mechanical Support of the Heart (also see Chapters 14 and 16)

Indications

In the setting of failure of dobutamine or vasodilator therapy to improve the hemodynamic status of the patient, and of the necessity for other catecholamine therapy to maintain a cardiac output and/or blood pressure, intraaortic balloon counterpulsation may be indicated. Mortality remains high (as noted in Chapter 16, surgical mortality subsequent to balloon dependence is very high).

Timing

In the patient with hypoperfusion and pulmonary congestion, no more than 1–2 hours of pharmacologic trial should be permitted (and then only with blood pressure being maintained at 90 mm Hg systolic by pressor agents), before a decision is made to proceed with intraaortic balloon counterpulsation.

Right Ventricular Infarction

Right ventricular infarction complicates transmural inferior or inferoposterior infarction in up to 35–40% of cases and presents characteristic clinical and hemodynamic findings that warrant prompt recognition to achieve optimal therapy.

At the bedside, patients exhibit hypotension, peripheral hypoperfusion, and jugular venous distention *not* associated with concomitant pulmonary congestion. Superficially, the physical signs of right ventricular infarction may resemble volume depletion (Forrester subset III) or true cardiogenic shock (Forrester subset IV).

The diagnosis is confirmed by right heart catheterization with a Swan-Ganz catheter. A distinct hemodynamic pattern resembling cardiac tamponade or constrictive pericarditis is observed. This includes elevated right atrial and right ventricular end-diastolic pressures, as well as elevated pulmonary arterial and PCW pressures. The demonstration of equalization of end-diastolic right heart chamber pressures in the setting of inferior infarction is virtually pathognomonic of this condition.

Treatment with intravascular volume expansion (crystalloid or colloid solutions) is mandatory. Since the infarcted right ventricle behaves as a passive conduit, systemic hypotension often persists until volume expansion increases the mean right atrial and/or PCW pressures to 15–20 mm of Hg. The concept of optimal fluid administration cannot be overemphasized.

Persistent hypotension unresponsive to volume expansion may require the additional use of sympathomimetic amines (dopamine, dobutamine), as previously detailed.

REFERENCES

Cohn JN, Franciosa JA: Vasodilator therapy of cardiac failure. N Engl J Med *297*:27 (Part 1), 254 (Part 2), 1977.

Forrester JS, Waters DD: Hospital treatment of congestive heart failure; Management according to hemodynamic profile. Am J Med *65*:173, 1978.

Sonnenblick EH, Fishman WH, LeJemtel TH: Dobutamine: A new synthetic cardioactive sympathetic amine. N Engl J Med *300*:17, 1979.

Tarazi RC: Sympathomimetic agents in the treatment of shock. Ann Intern Med *81*:364, 1974.

21

ACUTE MITRAL REGURGITATION AND RUPTURE OF THE INTERVENTRICULAR SEPTUM

Clinical Presentation of Mitral Regurgitation

Mitral regurgitation in the setting of coronary artery disease frequently is caused by either papillary muscle dysfunction or a left ventricular aneurysm. The diagnosis of mitral regurgitation is generally determined by auscultation of a systolic murmur at the left lower sternal border and cardiac apex—often with radiation to the axillary region. Transient mitral regurgitation may occur as a consequence of acute reversible *ischemia* and, as discussed later, can cause acute pulmonary edema. Typically, the appearance of mitral regurgitation, as a reflection of papillary muscle dysfunction, is hemodynamically unimportant since acute myocardial infarction frequently may compromise structural or functional integrity of the papillary muscle apparatus.

More important, however, is the severe form of mitral regurgitation, characterized as a loud systolic murmur associated with symptoms and signs of severe left ventricular failure developing in a patient with acute infarction, generally within the first week of hospitalization.

Three types of papillary muscle dysfunction may occur:

(1) *Papillary muscle dysfunction* as a consequence of myocardial ischemia involving either the anterolateral or posteromedial papillary muscle, resulting in acute left ventricular dysfunction, symptoms of chest pain with or without acute EKG changes, and overt congestive heart failure or pulmonary edema frequently. Because this mechanical sequela of myocardial infarction is often reversible, symptoms and signs of left ventricular dysfunction and electrocardiographic changes of ischemia may abate spontaneously or with the administration of vasodilators such as nitroglycerin. Frequently, the murmur of mitral regurgitation may wax and wane in this setting.

(2) Severe papillary muscle dysfunction may develop from the *rupture of one or two chordae tendineae,* which may produce severe left ventricular failure and significant acute mitral regurgitation. Similarly, rupture of one head of a papillary muscle generally produces hemodynamically severe mitral regurgitation, which may be responsive to initial medical treatment with inotropic agents, diuretics, and vasodilators. A prominent left-sided S4 gallop may be observed in patients with sinus rhythm from vigorous atrial contraction and a stiff, poorly compliant left ventricle. A systolic

parasternal lift may be appreciated at the lower left sternal border, and, of course, pulmonary congestion may be dramatic. (Hemodynamic findings will be discussed in detail later.)

(3) Patients who rupture an *entire papillary muscle* deteriorate rapidly and profoundly despite intensive medical management. The incidence of papillary muscle rupture observed at autopsy varies between 1 and 5% of cases. It occurs usually within the first 2 to 4 days following myocardial infarction. This catastrophic event is approximately 2.5 times as frequent in patients with inferior wall infarction as in those with anterior infarction. This difference in infarct location may relate, in part, to the dual blood supply of the anterolateral papillary muscle (left anterior descending and circumflex coronary arteries), in contrast to the single blood supply to the posteromedial papillary muscle from the right coronary artery. Thus, rupture of a posteromedial papillary muscle appears to have an anatomically worse prognosis. Rupture of an entire papillary muscle is heralded typically by the precipitous development of intractable pulmonary edema and shock. The physical findings are of "wide-open" mitral regurgitation with a loud holosystolic murmur and are otherwise identical to those just listed in section 2.

Mitral regurgitation secondary to papillary muscle dysfunction is frequently difficult to differentiate at the bedside from the murmur of ventricular septal rupture. The latter condition is typically associated with a harsh systolic murmur more localized to the left lower sternal border, with faint transmission to the cardiac apex and axilla. However, the traumatic "ventricular septal defect (VSD) murmur" may be indistinguishable on clinical grounds and diagnosis frequently requires insertion of a Swan-Ganz catheter.

Clinical Presentation of Ventricular Septal Rupture

Postinfarction ventricular septal defects may produce a systolic murmur maximal at the lower left sternal border, in contrast to the ruptured papillary muscle, in which the murmur is more localized to the left ventricular apex. A thrill may be found in either condition.

Ventricular septal rupture develops in 2% of hospitalized patients with acute myocardial infarction. The myocardial infarction responsible for ventricular septal rupture is usually transmural, is usually the patient's first infarction, and is located in the inferoposterior region of the left ventricle approximately 50% as often as it involves the anterior region. In contrast to patients who display rupture of the ventricular free wall following myocardial infarction, a prior history of hypertension is seen in only about 25% of patients with septal rupture. Ventricular septal rupture almost always occurs within 2 weeks of the onset of infarction, typically within the first week, and frequently is associated with new chest pain.

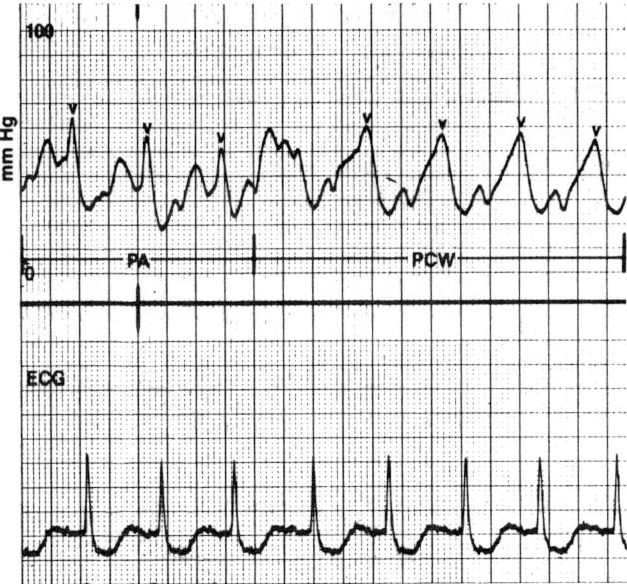

Figure 21–1. V waves in acute mitral regurgitation. V wave can be seen immediately following systolic pulmonary artery (PA) waveform, but it is more prominent on wedge (PCW) waveform. The second wave in the PA tracing can be identified as a V wave; it peaks at the same time following the R wave of the ECG (0.4 sec) as V wave on wedge tracing. Mean wedge pressure is higher than PA diastolic pressure. (From Kaye W: Textbook of Advanced Cardiac Life Support. Dallas, American Heart Association, 1981. Reproduced with permission.)

Diagnosis

Once *acute mitral regurgitation* or *ventricular septal rupture* is suspected, right heart catheterization at the bedside with a Swan-Ganz catheter should be performed. Ventricular septal rupture is confirmed by a "step up" in oxygen content in blood samples from the pulmonary artery compared with the right atrium. Giant "V" waves observed in the pulmonary capillary wedge pressure tracing are seen with acute mitral regurgitation secondary to papillary muscle and/or chordal rupture.

The protocol for performing the bedside differentiation of these two important mechanical complications of myocardial infarction follows:

(1) Pulmonary arterial and systemic arterial catheters are inserted, as discussed in Chapter 12. Serial duplicate blood samples (2 ml) should be obtained in heparinized syringes from superior vena cava, right atrium, right ventricle, and pulmonary artery as the balloon-tipped catheter is advanced into the pulmonary outflow tract. The samples should be free of air bubbles, and the catheters

should be capped and stored on ice until oximetry (quantitation of per cent oxygen saturation) can be performed.

(2) Once the PA catheter has been positioned in a distal pulmonary artery branch, the balloon should be inflated and a pulmonary capillary wedge pressure recorded. Typically, patients with severe mitral regurgitation will display a large "V" wave in the "wedge" tracing. While such a V wave is diagnostic of mitral regurgitation, occasional patients with septal rupture may exhibit prominent V waves in the wedge pressure recording because of functional mitral insufficiency (Fig. 21–1).

(3) To determine whether a patient has a significant oxygen step up, all blood samples obtained from the various locations just noted are analyzed for their oxygen content as follows:

Oxygen content of the sample in volumes % equals hemoglobin (grams per cent) × 1.39 × the per cent saturation of the sample. A difference of greater than 1 volume per cent between right atrial and right ventricular samples indicates a significant left-to-right shunt from an acquired VSD. The quantity of blood shunting left to right can be calculated according to the following formulae:

$$\text{Left-to-right shunt} = \text{pulmonary blood flow} - \text{systemic blood flow}$$

$$\text{Pulmonary blood flow} = \frac{\text{oxygen consumption}}{(\text{arterial blood } O_2 \text{ content}) - (\text{pulmonary arterial blood } O_2 \text{ content})}$$

$$\text{Systemic blood flow} = \frac{\text{oxygen consumption}}{(\text{arterial blood } O_2 \text{ content}) - (\text{right atrial blood } O_2 \text{ content})}$$

Oxygen consumption can be directly measured, or it can be calculated using an assumed oxygen consumption (140 ml O_2/M^2 body surface area).

Cineangiography should be performed preoperatively in all patients, since oxygen step ups at the pulmonary artery level have been reported to occur in the presence of acute severe mitral regurgitation owing to the massive reflux of oxygenated blood produced by the regurgitant wave.

Finally, these additional clinical features may aid in the differential diagnosis of partial papillary muscle rupture versus postinfarction VSD:

—Transmission of the murmur to the axilla is distinctly uncommon in interventricular septal rupture;

—ECG conduction disturbances are more frequently associated with septal rupture compared with papillary muscle rupture;

—VSD is a more frequent complication than papillary muscle rupture in anterior infarction; in contrast, papillary muscle rupture is more common with inferior infarction.

Course and Treatment

The medical management of both acute mitral regurgitation and ventricular septal rupture is similar. Therapy is aimed at attempts to compensate the "volume-overloaded" left ventricle until cardiac catheterization and surgical repair can be attempted.

Mild-to-modest mitral regurgitation and VSD produce left ventricular failure, which may be amenable to a combination of digitalis, diuretics, and vasodilator therapy. (See Chapters 19 and 20.)

In patients with a pulmonary capillary wedge (PCW) pressure of greater than 25 mm Hg and a cardiac index of less than 2.2 L/min/M^2 (Forrester subset IV), more aggressive management with parenteral vasodilators is indicated:

(1) A nitroprusside infusion should be initiated in the presence of intraarterial systemic pressure monitoring. An initial infusion rate of 0.5 μg/Kg/min (approximately 35 μg/min) should be initiated and the infusion rate increased at 5 minute intervals until the PCW pressure falls below 18 mm Hg. Systolic arterial pressure should not be permitted to fall below 95 mm Hg. If nitroprusside is not sufficient to reduce the PCW pressure or if systemic hypotension precludes its use, intravenous nitroglycerin should be employed, at an infusion rate beginning at 0.5 μg/kg/min (approximately 35 μg/min). This infusion should be increased every 3 to 5 minutes until PCW pressure falls below 18 mm Hg.

(2) If a patient is hypotensive in the face of an elevated PCW, inotropic support with a synthetic sympathomimetic amine is indicated. Either dopamine or dobutamine may raise systemic arterial pressure and, more importantly, cardiac output. The dose for these agents is similar to that employed for cardiogenic shock (see Chapter 20). Evidence now suggests that the combined use of inotropic and vasodilator agents may be more beneficial than either agent used alone for decreasing afterload and augmenting forward cardiac output. Thus, dopamine or dobutamine in combination with nitroprusside is a favorable synergistic combined therapy for severe cardiac failure following acute mitral regurgitation or traumatic septal rupture.

However, it is important to emphasize that even combined inotropic-vasodilator pharmacologic therapy is generally unsuccessful in patients with wide-open mitral regurgitation secondary to a partially ruptured papillary muscle head or traumatic VSD, since approximately 60% of these patients develop cardiogenic shock. The medical management of the cardiogenic shock syndrome is dismal (see Chapter 20), but, unlike cardiogenic shock secondary to left ventricular damage, many patients with septal rupture or mitral regurgitation have intact ventricular function and thus have a purely *mechanical* cause for their acute cardiac failure. Accordingly, the most physiologic support for these patients is intraaortic balloon counterpulsation followed by cardiac surgical repair.

(3) Intraaortic balloon counterpulsation (IABC) may be potentially life-saving in patients with either of these two severe complications of myocardial infarction. IABC diminishes afterload by facilitating ventricular emptying during systole and augments retrograde coronary perfusion during diastole. Thus, in the presence of left ventricular dysfunction due to *mechanical* consequences of myocardial infarction, IABC augments myocardial oxygen supply and diminishes oxygen demand. The availability of newer percutaneous IABC devices permits the bedside application of this technique to critically ill patients. The major contraindication to IABC is severe obliterative peripheral vascular disease.

Once IABC is instituted, left ventriculography, coronary angiography, and subsequent operation should be performed without delay since improvement secondary to balloon pumping is often temporary.

(4) Operative management for closure of a ventricular septal rupture, or acute mitral valve replacement with or without myocardial revascularization, remains the only viable therapeutic option. Ideally, cardiac surgery is postponed until the patient is over the acute phase of myocardial infarction, but this rarely can be accomplished. More commonly, patients with intact ventricular function can be salvaged by emergency catheterization and surgical intervention. Nevertheless, even in the most experienced surgical hands, such operations carry significant morbidity and mortality.

REFERENCES

Braunwald E: Mitral regurgitation: Physiologic, clinical and surgical considerations. N Engl J Med *281*:425, 1969.

Daggett WM, Guyton RA, Mundth ED, et al: Surgery for post-myocardial infarct ventricular septal defect. Ann Surg *186*:260, 1976.

Gunnar RM, Loeb HS: Shock in acute myocardial infarction: Evolution of physiologic therapy. J Am Coll Cardiol *1*:154, 1983.

Montoya A, McKeever L, Scanlon P, et al: Early repair of ventricular septal rupture after infarction. Am J Cardiol *45*:345, 1980.

Radford MJ, Johnson RA, Daggett WM, et al: Ventricular septal rupture: A review of clinical and physiologic features and an analysis of survival. Circulation *64*:545, 1981.

Richard C, Ricome CL, Rimailho A, et al: Combined hemodynamic effects of dopamine and dobutamine in cardiogenic shock. Circulation *67*:620, 1982.

Wei JY, Hutchins GM, Bulkley BH: Papillary muscle rupture in fatal acute myocardial infarction—a potentially treatable form of cardiogenic shock. Ann Intern Med *90*:149, 1979.

22
MISCELLANEOUS COMPLICATIONS POSTMYOCARDIAL INFARCTION

PERICARDITIS

Pericarditis complicating acute myocardial infarction occurs in approximately 10 to 15 percent of patients, as judged by the clinical finding of a pericardial friction rub, although data obtained from postmortem studies suggest that the true incidence may be considerably higher. In general, pericarditis is associated with transmural infarction with concomitant inflammation of contiguous pericardium and may occur as commonly in inferior or posterior infarction as in anterior infarction.

The time course of pericarditis complicating myocardial infarction is variable, but a friction rub is most common on the second and third days after the onset of myocardial necrosis and may be present for up to 1 week following myocardial infarction. It is rare for simple pericarditis to occur within the first 24 hours following infarction or later than 1 week.

The appearance of pericarditis remote from an acute initial ischemic event raises the suspicion of autoimmune pleuropericarditis (Dressler's syndrome, discussed later).

Clinical Features

The classic physical finding of postinfarction pericarditis is a three-component friction rub associated with symptoms of pleuritic chest discomfort, low-grade fever or leukocytosis. The pericardial friction rub is frequently transient, and, unless the patient's chest is auscultated serially during the first few days following myocardial infarction, it is frequently missed. The pericardial friction rub's three components relate to atrial systole, ventricular contraction, and the early phase of ventricular diastolic filling. Best results are obtained with firm pressure of the diaphragm chest piece of the stethoscope against the anterior chest wall, with the patient supine. The pericardial friction rub may attenuate in the sitting position and frequently is monophasic or biphasic. It may be difficult to distinguish from a systolic murmur, although the pericardial friction rub in general has a scratchy, high-pitched, close-to-the-ear, auscultatory quality.

The appearance of pericarditis may often confuse the clinical picture in the early phase of acute myocardial infarction because of the appearance of chest pain, electrocardiographic ST-T wave abnormalities, and the evanescent auscultatory findings. Chest pain is not an infrequent complaint during the first few days following admission to the Coronary Care Unit, and the development of chest discomfort following myocardial infarction raises the suspicion of infarct extension or unstable angina (see Chapter 23). In pericarditis, the chest pain is generally atypical in location, site, distribution, and duration but frequently may mimic pain of ischemic origin.

Diagnosis

Because the diagnosis is seldom entertained in the absence of a pericardial friction rub, it is easy to understand why the presentation may be difficult to distinguish from that of ongoing myocardial ischemia.

Similarly, the electrocardiogram may show ST segment elevation and/or T wave inversion, which may be difficult to distinguish from infarct extension or ischemia. In general, however, pericarditis produces global repolarization abnormalities without a predilection for segmental location, and when these changes occur in the absence of serum enzyme elevations compatible with further myocardial necrosis, the diagnosis of pericarditis becomes more secure. Additionally, P-R segment depression has been described as a sensitive marker for pericarditis, although this is not universally seen. Moreover, tachycardia is frequently associated with pericarditis as well as myocardial ischemia and may further complicate the clinical picture. Finally, postinfarct pericarditis may be confused with pulmonary embolism or pneumonia.

Unlike infectious etiologies of pericarditis, postinfarct pericarditis is not often associated with significant pericardial effusion, thus echocardiography is not an extremely useful diagnostic aid. However, in some cases, an enlarging cardiac silhouette and/or ultrasonic evidence for pericardial effusion may be delineated by noninvasive means.

Course and Treatment

Treatment is directed more toward symptomatic relief than toward interrupting the inflammatory process, which is generally transitory and self-limited. A pericardial friction rub is said to be associated with a higher incidence of congestive heart failure and arrhythmias (particularly supraventricular arrhythmias), but the medical literature does not support the thesis that these contribute to increased mortality following myocardial infarction. Moreover, it is unclear whether treatment with antiinflammatory agents in any way influences the course of postinfarction pericarditis.

The simplest and most effective agent remains oral salicylates (650 mg po q 4–6 hr). If patients do not respond to salicylates or have a medical contraindication to salicylate therapy, other nonsteroidal antiinflammatory agents such as ibuprofen or indomethacin may be used. Ibuprofen is employed in doses ranging from 300–400 mg every 6–8 hours, and indomethacin is generally administered in doses of 25–50 mg every 6 hours. When salicylates or nonsteroidal antiinflammatory agents are ineffective for severe, prolonged postinfarction pericarditis, corticosteroids may be employed, although prolonged therapy should be avoided since some evidence suggests that it may result in aneurysm formation—and possibly myocardial rupture—owing to impaired scar formation and delayed healing postinfarction. We do not recommend the use of corticosteroids except in extreme symptomatic cases.

Finally, in individuals with pericarditis who display increased supraventricular ectopy, we favor the prophylactic administration of digoxin to prevent atrial fibrillation. It has been shown that pericarditis-induced atrial ectopy may presage atrial fibrillation, and the judicious use of modest amounts of digoxin (0.25 mg po bid × 2 days, then 0.25 mg po every day) may be efficacious in preventing supraventricular tachycardia.

DRESSLER'S SYNDROME

Dressler's syndrome is a clinical entity characterized by pericarditis, pleurisy, fever, leukocytosis, and pulmonary infiltrates that may appear 1 week to several months following acute myocardial infarction. The incidence of this complication is uncertain, but it may occur in up to 4% of patients following myocardial infarction. The etiology is unclear, although autoimmune mechanisms, with or without a supervening viral infection, are presumed to be causative. Certain patients have been shown to exhibit antiheart antibodies, although this is not a universal finding. Dressler's syndrome shares many common features with the postcardiotomy syndrome, posttraumatic pericarditis, and recurrent idiopathic pericarditis. A common denominator appears to be myocardial injury with associated blood in the pericardial cavity that may provide the inflammatory basis for this disorder. The histology of the pericardium may be normal or may show nonspecific inflammatory reaction with fibrinous exudate.

Clinical Features

A considerable amount of overlap appears between pericarditis in the course of acute myocardial infarction and Dressler's syndrome. Certainly, the time course may be indistinguishable following acute infarction, although in general Dressler's syndrome occurs late in the course of acute infarction. Both pericardial and pleural pain may be present and may be difficult to distinguish from the pain of acute infarction. However, the pain is generally aggravated by inspiration or coughing, is relieved by sitting, and frequently radiates to the scapular region.

Fevers as high as 40°C have been reported, and both pleural and pericardial rubs are heard on auscultation—the latter may be transitory in the majority of patients and may frequently be missed. Signs of pleural effusion may be demonstrable, and the chest roentgenogram may show pleural effusions or pulmonary infiltrates localized at the bases. An enlarged cardiac silhouette caused by pericardial effusion may be seen in three fifths of patients.

The electrocardiogram shows changes consistent with pericarditis, with diffuse ST segment elevations, T wave inversions, and, rarely, electrical alternans. Clearly, the clinical features of Dressler's syndrome may be confused with infarct extension or recurrence but most often can be distinguished from these entities by the absence of new electrocardiographic Q waves and concomitant cardiac enzyme elevations.

Diagnosis

There are no specific positive laboratory studies in Dressler's syndrome. There may be evidence for leukocytosis, and frequently there is evidence of elevated erythrocyte sedimentation rate. The presence of fever, pleuritic chest pain, and pericardial and/or pleural effusion in the setting of recent myocardial infarction supports the diagnosis of Dressler's syndrome.

Course and Treatment

Dressler's syndrome is usually self-limited and treatment is nonspecific. If patients are symptomatic from pleuropericarditis, aspirin, indomethacin, and other nonsteroidal antiinflammatory agents may be effective in hastening the resolution of the syndrome. In rare instances, corticosteroid therapy may be necessary. It is emphasized that antiinflammatory agents are generally proscribed in patients who are taking concomitant anticoagulant therapy, owing to the increased incidence of gastrointestinal bleeding and potential intrapericardial bleeding.

Occasionally, recurrent subacute episodes of Dressler's syndrome may occur, and chronic pericardial effusions have been reported to develop. In these individuals, the syndrome may last from months to even years, and such refractory cases may require multiple courses of corticosteroid therapy. In general, prednisone, 60 mg/24 hr, is administered until symptoms and signs have abated, usually within 4 to 7 days. Subsequently, the dose is tapered and maintained until clinical manifestations have been completely suppressed.

PULMONARY EMBOLISM

Clinical Features

Pulmonary embolism may complicate myocardial infarction in one of two ways:

(1) as a complication of deep venous thrombosis of the lower extremities;

(2) as a complication of atrial or ventricular mural thrombosis.

The exact incidence of pulmonary embolism complicating myocardial infarction is uncertain. Historically, embolic complications of myocardial infarction were reported to be as high as 15 to 20%, and, undoubtedly, this reflects the protracted bedrest that attended the medical management of myocardial infarction up through the early 1960s. Accordingly, the use of anticoagulants (heparin and/or coumadin) has been advocated by many as a prophylactic measure for patients with myocardial infarction, although detailed prospective data in support of this concept are lacking.

Another consideration regarding pulmonary embolism relates to the initial differential diagnosis of chest pain on admission to the CCU. While the clinical presentation of pulmonary embolism is frequently associated with chest pain, dyspnea, diaphoresis, anxiety, tachycardia, and/or atrial or ventricular arrhythmias, often it may pose considerable difficulties in the differential diagnosis of acute chest pain, since it may mimic acute coronary insufficiency or myocardial infarction. In addition, the electrocardiogram may reveal a myriad of changes that are nonspecific for either myocardial infarction or pulmonary embolism.

Following admission to the CCU, the patient at bedrest is known to be at higher risk for developing deep venous thrombosis of the lower extremities. It is not surprising that stasis induced by the immobility during the early stage of confinement to the CCU may predispose certain individuals to venous thrombosis, particularly those with left ventricular failure, obesity, varicosities, or prior history of thromboembolism.

In such a setting, patients with known cardiac disease who display an unexplained clinical deterioration characterized by acute atrial arrhythmia, worsening dyspnea and/or hypoxemia, or the rapid development of congestive heart failure may indeed have pulmonary embolism as an explanation for such decompensation.

Diagnosis

Pulmonary embolism is a difficult diagnosis to establish, since laboratory and noninvasive tests are frequently nondiagnostic.

Arterial hypoxemia on a room air arterial blood gas sample, in a patient without left ventricular failure, may raise the suspicion of pulmonary embolism. If an embolism is suspected on clinical grounds, and if the patient's condition permits, a lung scan should be performed. Mobile cameras are available to perform this study at the bedside in many hospitals, and, even when they are not, a strong suspicion warrants transfer of the patient to the Nuclear Medicine or Radiology department to obtain the study. A negative perfusion scan virtually excludes a significant pulmonary embolus. A positive scan, with multiple segmental or subsegmental perfusion defects, supports the diagnosis but is not diagnostic. If more diagnostic specificity is desired, a ventilation-perfusion scan (if available) may help delineate a ventilation-perfusion mismatch and thus further aid in the predictive accuracy of the test. Pulmonary angiography is performed in clinical situations in which the highest degree of diagnostic accuracy is required, when alteration in therapy depends on an established diagnosis.

Adjunctive diagnostic procedures, such as ^{131}I radiolabeled fibrinogen leg scanning or impedance plethysmography, may aid in the identification of an embolic source in the lower extremities.

Fibrin degradation products may be elevated in patients with significant pulmonary embolism but are a nonspecific finding that may be elevated in a variety of conditions, including myocardial infarction.

The ECG may show a variety of abnormalities, including right axis shift, acute right bundle branch block, right atrial enlargement, or an S_1-Q_3-T_3 pattern indicative of "right heart strain." More typically, however, the ECG will reveal only nonspecific repolarization abnormalities. Thus, the ECG is usually an insensitive indicator of pulmonary embolism.

Course and Treatment

Pulmonary embolism, if confirmed by radionuclide imaging techniques and/or pulmonary arteriography, should be treated with "full-dose" heparin in all patients in whom there is no clinical contraindication.

Two protocols for heparin administration are suitable.

(1) If continuous intravenous heparin administration is desired, an initial loading dose of 5000 to 10,000 units is given as a bolus injection, followed by an infusion of between 500 to 1000 units/hr, the dose being adjusted on the basis of an activated partial thromboplastin time (PTT) determined at periodic intervals. A value of 60 to 80 seconds (or twice the control PTT) is considered therapeutic.

(2) If intermittent intravenous heparin administration is desired, the usual dosage is 5000 units q 4 hr, although it is recognized that the dose may vary from 2500 to 10,000 units among various individuals. Again, the efficacy of therapy should be verified by serial PTT determinations.

Heparin therapy should be continued for a minimum of 7 to 10 days—the time interval required for stabilization of the thrombus within the venous circulation. At this time, the concurrent administration of oral warfarin should be initiated, and treatment with both heparin and warfarin should overlap for approximately 3 to 5 days to permit an adequate antithrombin effect from the oral agent. Oral warfarin therapy should be administered for at least 3 months.

Minidose heparin (subcutaneous heparin, 5000 to 10,000 units q 12 hr) is *not* suitable therapy for pulmonary embolism. Its only use is for deep venous thrombosis prophylaxis.

If a patient has a life-threatening contraindication to intravenous heparin, alternatives to anticoagulation include vena caval interruption procedures.

SYSTEMIC EMBOLISM

Clinical Features

Mural thrombi may complicate extensive transmural infarctions and less commonly subendocardial infarctions. They may also occur as a sequela of ventricular aneurysms, most notably in patients with apical dyskinesis following a transmural anterior wall myocardial infarction (MI). Mural thrombi may form at the site of endocardial injury and may be expelled into the systemic circulation as emboli. This complication appears to be infrequent, although its effects may be devastating, resulting in stroke and organ infarction or acute arterial insufficiency of an extremity. Such peripheral embolization to the cerebral or systemic circulation generally occurs within weeks to months following an acute myocardial infarction. Such individuals may exhibit symptoms and signs of a transient ischemic attack or stroke and may show classic focal neurologic findings.

Other individuals may exhibit abrupt arterial insufficiency in one or both lower extremities. The classic clinical presentation of such a peripheral embolism involves the five "Ps": pallor, pain, paralysis, paresthesias, and pulselessness.

Diagnosis

The diagnosis of systemic embolism, as outlined, is predicated on clinical findings of either focal neurologic deficit or the sudden onset of a cold extremity or digit. Embolism to the central nervous system mandates prompt clinical attention. If available, computed tomography (CT scan) should be obtained as soon as possible. Alternatively, a lumbar puncture to exclude the presence or absence of hemorrhage or xanthochromia in the spinal fluid may aid in the decision concerning anticoagulation. The neurology service should be consulted without delay.

When the diagnosis of peripheral embolism has been made, full-dose heparin therapy should be instituted at once and the vascular surgical service should be promptly notified. Diagnostic arteriography is generally performed under local anesthesia, and an embolectomy using a Fogarty catheter is frequently successful in promoting limb salvage.

MYOCARDIAL RUPTURE

Clinical Presentation

Rupture of the left ventricular free wall is the third most common fatal complication of myocardial infarction, following arrhythmias and cardiogenic shock (pump failure). This complication occurs in approximately 10% of fatal myocardial infarctions. It is most common in elderly females, with a peak incidence occurring in the 8th decade. It is more frequently encountered with first infarctions, occurring during the first week (generally 2 to 4 days) after transmural infarction. Systemic hypertension in patients who subsequently develop myocardial rupture appears frequently in the history.

Four clinical patterns may emerge:

(1) Patients will complain of recurrent prolonged chest pain during the first few days postinfarction, followed by profound dyspnea, hypotension, and neck vein distention with rapid progression to electromechanical dissociation (EMD) and death.

(2) Less commonly, patients may have a subacute onset of features suggesting cardiac tamponade over a period of hours. Pulsus paradoxus, distended neck veins, tachycardia, and systemic hypotension may subsequently ensue. When the paradox is greater than 20 mm Hg, there is frequently a diminutive peripheral pulse by palpation.

(3) Formation of a left ventricular pseudoaneurysm may presage cardiac rupture. The left ventricular pseudoaneurysm actually represents an incompletely contained cardiac rupture that is frequently connected to the left ventricular chamber through an isthmus. Thus, the pseudoaneurysm comprises organized clot and fibrous tissue, in contrast to the true ventricular aneurysm that contains endocardial, myocardial, and epicardial elements. The continuous movement of blood back and forth through the neck of the aneurysm may produce systolic and/or diastolic murmurs.

(4) Electromechanical dissociation may be the presenting feature of cardiac rupture, with a sudden loss of consciousness, associated with a normal cardiac rhythm by ECG but without palpable pulse or audible heart sounds. In this subset of patients, few clinical symptoms may antedate myocardial rupture.

Diagnosis

The diagnosis of cardiac rupture, as just outlined, is predicated on the clinical recognition of this potential complication in the first week following myocardial infarction. Thus, any patient who has an *unexplained,* profound deterioration of hemodynamics is a likely candidate for this mechanical complication. Although death usually occurs within minutes, some patients (particularly those with cardiac tamponade or pseudoaneurysm) may be noninvasively imaged with an echocardiogram (M-mode or 2D) to determine significant pericardial fluid or abnormal ("swinging") septal motion. Insertion of a Swan-Ganz catheter at the bedside may confirm diastolic equilibration of intracardiac filling pressures indicative of cardiac tamponade.

Course and Treatment

Cardiac rupture is a medical emergency. If patients can be stabilized and supported hemodynamically with intraaortic balloon counterpulsation, they should be transferred to the operating room where the defect can be closed.

Despite heroic attempts, the prognosis for cardiac rupture is very grave.

REFERENCES

Biorck G, Mogensen L, Nyquist O, et al: Studies of myocardial rupture with cardiac tamponade in acute myocardial infarction. Chest *61*:4, 1973.

Bulkley BH, Roberts WC: Steroid therapy during acute myocardial infarction: A cause of delayed healing and of ventricular aneurysm. Am J Med *56*:244, 1974.

Dressler W: The post-myocardial infarction syndrome: A report of 44 cases. Arch Intern Med *103*:28, 1956.

Goldman LR, Feinstein AR: Anticoagulants and myocardial infarction. Ann Intern Med *84*:700, 1976.

Lichstein E, Liu H, Gupta P: Pericarditis complicating acute myocardial infarction: Incidence of complications and significance of ECG on admission. Am Heart J *87*:246, 1974.

Miarchos AP, McKendrich CS: Prognosis of pericarditis after acute myocardial infarction. Br Heart J *35*:49, 1973.

Spodick DH: Acute Pericarditis. New York, Grune & Stratton, 1959.

Spodick DH: Pericardial Diseases. Philadelphia, FA Davis, 1976.

23

POSTINFARCTION ANGINA

Definition

Postinfarction angina is characterized by precordial discomfort that has the usual anginal characteristics or is similar in character to the symptoms present at the time of the patient's acute myocardial infarction (MI).

It typically occurs within 21 days of the acute MI.

It presents as a new episode following a pain-free interval or as an episode following mild residual pain within the first 24 hours following infarction.

Accompanying transient ST elevation or depression or T wave changes are helpful in establishing the diagnosis, but these may be minimal or absent.

Recurrent enzyme elevation is absent, although infrequent or sporadic sampling may not detect myocardial necrosis due to an extension.

Initial Medical Treatment

The treatment is similar to that given to the patient with unstable angina who has not suffered an acute myocardial infarction. However, since the patient with a recent infarction has a compromised myocardium, treatment must be given with greater care and under closer observation to avoid any detrimental effect on hemodynamics.

(1) Treat the acute episode with sublingual nitroglycerin.

(2) Eliminate any inciting events, such as activity, emotional stress.

(3) Treat heart failure, if present, to reduce myocardial oxygen demand.

(4) Unless postinfarction angina is clearly due to (2) or (3), prophylactic pharmacologic therapy should be initiated:

Isosorbide dinitrate (ISD). Begin with 10 mg po; in 4 hours increase to 20–30 mg and repeat every 4 hours thereafter. If headaches are severe, dosage may have to be decreased.

Nitroglycerin paste may be used in place of ISD. Begin with 0.5 inch; in 4 hours increase to 1 inch and repeat every 4 hours thereafter. Doses up to 2 inches every 4 hours may be needed, if anginal symptoms persist.

Propranolol. Begin with 10 mg; in 4 hours increase to 20 mg and repeat every 6 hours. In patients without signs of failure (and with frequent clinical observations), increase to 40 mg every 6 hours.

For Recurrent Anginal Episodes

(1) Increase ISD to 30 mg and then to 40 mg, if tolerated.

(2) If nitroglycerin paste is being used, increase to 1.5 inches and then to 2 inches, if tolerated.

(3) Increase the dose of propranolol, depending on the clinical status of the patient. If the resting heart rate remains above 60 and signs of heart failure are absent, increasing to 60 mg q 6 hr with frequent clinical observations is a safe and additionally efficacious therapy.

(4) Further recurrence of pain while the patient is in the CCU may be treated with additional increases of beta-blockade and nitrates. If pain episodes continue to be severe and frequent, the institution of intravenous nitroglycerin frequently provides prompt relief, with the added safety of rapid adjustment of dose should hypotension occur or an increase be necessary.

Whether coronary spasm is a prominent part of this syndrome is a matter of debate at present. Episodes associated with ST elevation that occur without provocation while the patient is at bedrest are highly suspect. The treatment of choice in such a situation is a primary vasodilator (intravenous nitroglycerin, oral or cutaneous nitroglycerin) or calcium channel blocker (nifedipine or diltiazem). The particular drug and route of administration are dictated by the severity of the pain. Protocols for the use of intravenous nitroglycerin and nifedipine or diltiazem are listed in Chapter 17.

Refractory Angina

Pain poorly responsive to medical therapy represents a medical emergency. It is best treated by insertion of an intraaortic balloon pump (IABP), which generally results in prompt cessation of episodes of pain in the majority of cases. Cardiac catheterization should be carried out once stabilization has occurred and can be expected to demonstrate high-grade occlusive coronary disease. In most patients, stabilization will be maintained and the IABP can be discontinued; surgery for those with left main coronary or "left main equivalent" disease can then be deferred for 4–6 weeks. Others who cannot be weaned from the balloon without recurrence of angina will require earlier surgery.

Recurrent Angina Post-CCU

Recurrence of pain in the post-CCU period during increased activity should be treated with increasing beta-blockade and nitrates, as indicated. Cardiac catheterization is usually required during the period of hospitalization; in most cases coronary bypass surgery, if indicated, can be safely postponed until 3 months postinfarction, although the angiographic demonstration of critical coronary lesions may mandate urgent myocardial revascularization within days to weeks of an initial myocardial infarction.

REFERENCES

Brundage BH, Ullyot DJ, Winokur S, et al: The role of aortic balloon pumping in post infarction angina—a different perspective. Circulation *62*(Suppl 1):119, 1980.

Dawson JT, Hall RJ, Hallman GL, et al: Mortality in patients undergoing coronary artery bypass after myocardial infarction. Am J Cardiol *33*:483, 1974.

Weintraub RM, Aroesty JM, Paulin S, et al: Medically refractory unstable angina pectoris. I. Long-term follow-up of patients undergoing intraaortic balloon counterpulsation and operation. Am J Cardiol *43*:877, 1979.

24

SALVAGE OF ISCHEMIC MYOCARDIUM AND LIMITATION OF INFARCT SIZE

Rationale

Supply/Demand (See Chapter 2)

The acute infarct area consists of necrotic and ischemic but still viable cells. It is believed that a large proportion of these ischemic cells become necrotic during the acute course of infarction. Measures that improve the myocardial oxygen supply/demand relationship have the potential for maintaining the viability of these cells, thus decreasing the amount of infarcted myocardium and improving the ability of the heart to function as a pump.

Previous Studies

Extensive animal experimentation has demonstrated that reductions in myocardial infarction size can be achieved using a variety of approaches. Application to humans, however, is limited by several factors:

The amount of salvageable myocardium decreases rapidly. For all practical purposes, interventions must be instituted within 4–6 hours from the onset of infarction;

Studies to substantiate the validity of the animal findings in humans have been severely limited by the inability to make serial clinical measurements of infarct size easily; and

The long-term outcome of interventions in humans is not known. Each intervention has associated undesirable effects. In addition, the eventual status of the "salvaged" myocardium remains undetermined; specific concerns that heterogeneous ischemic and normal myocardium ("the border zone") may be a site for serious arrhythmias or recurrent angina are presently unanswered and await the outcome of several studies now in progress.

Approaches

Improvements in Myocardial Oxygen Supply

Improving Blood Flow in the Affected Coronary Artery

Acute Coronary Thrombolysis. Although coronary thrombosis has been hypothesized to be a result rather than a cause of acute myocardial infarction, many patients catheterized in the acute situation are reported to have coronary obstruction owing to blood clot formation. In some studies, improvements in myocardial contraction patterns have been seen following clot removal, either by mechanical means (catheter guide wire) or with thrombolytic agents. Streptokinase is currently the most widely used agent of this class. When infused directly into the coronary artery, streptokinase results in dissolution of clot in approximately 70% of patients in whom lytic therapy is administered early in the course of infarction.

Two recent trials evaluating the efficacy of *intracoronary* fibrinolytic therapy in acute myocardial infarction are available for review. Goldstein and coworkers performed a randomized placebo-controlled trial with intracoronary streptokinase administered to 40 patients within 6 hours of their hospitalization. Coronary reperfusion was established in 60% of treated patients, but there was no statistically significant improvement in left ventricular function, as measured by serial radionuclide ejection fraction, up to 5 months after initial therapy.

Conversely, Andersen et al, using a similar protocol but administering the intracoronary streptokinase within the first 3 hours of presentation, showed that coronary perfusion was re-established in 80% of treated patients and was associated with a significant improvement in serial radionuclide ejection fraction, Killip class, and decreased time to peak plasma cardiac enzyme concentration. This study indicated that early (≤ 3 hours) intracoronary fibrinolytic therapy had a beneficial effect on the early course of acute myocardial infarction. Thus, the time course of early streptokinase administration may promote myocardial salvage in some patients with acute myocardial infarction, but additional controlled large-scale studies are needed to confirm these preliminary observations.

Studies investigating streptokinase use by *intravenous* infusion have shown a significant reduction in 6 month mortality but have been attended by bleeding complications. While promising, this treatment remains investigational, with studies of its use in acute myocardial infarction confined to a few centers. It remains an experimental approach with great promise.

Acute Percutaneous Transluminal Coronary Angioplasty (PTCA). PTCA during the acute phase of myocardial infarction remains a controversial and experimental procedure. A recent report (Myer et al) has demonstrated its efficacy and safety within the first 8 hours after the onset of symptoms and following the use of intracoronary streptokinase for thrombolysis.

Acute Coronary Bypass Surgery. This modality usually has been reserved for emergency situations in patients with in-hospital infarctions. A recent report by Berg et al has shown that it can be performed routinely on patients within 6 hours of the acute infarction with a combined operative and 1 year mortality of 3.2%, and a decrease in postinfarction angina and aneurysm formation. Acute surgical intervention remains an experimental approach confined to institutions with sufficient resources and manpower to ensure the immediate availability of the surgical team around the clock.

Pharmacologic Improvement in Myocardial Perfusion. Nitroglycerin has been shown to improve the blood flow to ischemic portions of the endocardium, presumably by increasing coronary collateral blood flow. This effect is disputed by some investigators and is probably of lesser importance than its effects in reducing myocardial demand (described later).

Mechanical Improvement in Coronary Flow. Intraaortic balloon counterpulsation can reduce the extent of myocardial ischemia in humans as measured by the extent of ST segment elevation. It presumably does so by improving diastolic coronary blood flow, as well as by reducing afterload (and thus myocardial oxygen demand). It is not clear which of these alternatives predominates. Although the newer percutaneous placement technique permits rapid insertion, the complexities of counterpulsation use, the potential hazards to the patient, and the limitation of medical resources make this a less than ideal intervention for use in the routine situation.

Direct Increases in Oxygenation. The use of 100% oxygen administration by mask will reduce the amount of ischemic myocardium, as measured by the degree of ST segment elevation. This provides a rationale for the routine administration of oxygen to the patient with acute MI. Whether lower inspired oxygen concentrations, i.e., by nasal cannulae that are less disturbing to the patient, will be similarly efficacious must await further studies.

Improved Oxygen Diffusion. Administration of IV hyaluronidase is accompanied by a decrease in ischemia during acute MI (as measured by the extent of ST segment elevation). The mechanism of action is unclear but is thought to be a facilitation of oxygen transport through the interstitial spaces. Administration may be associated with allergic reaction (local or systemic) and requires prior testing. No large studies have yet verified the usefulness of this modality, although the results will be forthcoming soon of a large, multicenter trial on Myocardial Infarction Limitation of Infarct Size (MILIS), which is investigating the potential utility of hyaluronidase.

Mannitol. Although originally described as decreasing cell swelling during the ischemia of acute MI, mannitol seems to have its major application during prolonged coronary artery occlusion and as a cardioplegic solution in coronary artery bypass surgery.

Decrease in Myocardial Oxygen Demand

Beta-Blockade with Selective and Nonselective Beta-Blockers. By reducing heart rate and myocardial contractility (both major determinants of demand), myocardial oxygen requirements are markedly reduced. Patients dependent on myocardial beta-stimulation for maintenance of cardiac function will experience an abrupt onset of cardiac decompensation on propranolol administration. Therefore it must be given with extreme caution and never to a patient with compromised cardiovascular function (unless appropriate hemodynamic parameters are being followed). Its effect in reducing acute infarct size in humans has not been verified in a large study, although several large-scale postinfarction trials have verified the efficary of beta-blockers in secondary infarct prophylaxis and reduction of mortality.

Pharmacologic Reductions of Preload and Afterload. Nitroglycerin has been seen to improve ST segment elevation clinically in the acute MI patient and, by inference, the extent of myocardial ischemia. As noted, some improvement in blood flow into the ischemic area is thought to occur, but the major physiologic effect is on the peripheral circulation to decrease myocardial oxygen demand. Care must be taken to insure that blood pressure does not fall appreciably (resulting in a reduced coronary blood flow) or heart rate increase reflexly (resulting in an increase in myocardial oxygen demand). Its use in the treatment of ischemic pain during acute MI constitutes a major recent innovation in coronary care; its use in the absence of pain remains experimental. Use of nitroprusside as an afterload reducing agent has been shown to increase the extent or severity of the infarction. In the absence of hypertension or overt congestive heart failure, it should not be given in acute myocardial infarction.

Reduction in Heart Size. Cardiac dilation increases oxygen demands. Thus heart failure, if appropriately treated, can reduce demand and thus reduce infarct size. Agents that reduce preload (such as diuretics) represent the most effective therapy for the treatment of uncomplicated heart failure in the acute MI patient. Positive inotropic agents, including digitalis, will always increase oxygen demand but are efficacious if they simultaneously reduce demand by decreasing heart size. Thus they should not be given in the absence of cardiac dilation.

Other Approaches

Cellullar Lysosomal Stabilization. The use of adrenocorticosteroids has been experimentally shown to reduce infarct size, presumably by stabilizing lysosomal membranes and preventing release of their cell-damaging contents. Ventricular rupture in the postinfarct period of patients on long-term steroid therapy has been reported; thus, use of adrenocorticosteroids to limit infarct size must await further studies.

Clinical Use

No proved modality reduces infarct size in humans. Most approaches are limited by the inability to treat the patient early after clinical presentation or by potential or recognized adverse effects. At the present time, routine coronary care, which by its very nature reduces oxygen demand, remains the mainstay of this approach. Other modalities must be considered experimental at present.

REFERENCES

Anderson JL, Marshall HW, Bray BE, et al: A randomized trial of intracoronary streptokinase in the treatment of acute myocardial infarction. N Engl J Med *308*:1312, 1983.

Bache RJ: Effect of nitroglycerin and arterial hypertension on myocardial blood flow during acute coronary occlusion in the dog. Circulation *57*:557, 1978.

Berg JR, Selinger SL, Leonard JJ, et al: Immediate coronary artery bypass for acute evolving myocardial infarction. J Thorac Cardiovasc Surg *81*:493, 1981.

Chiariello M, Gold HK, Leinbach MD, et al: Comparison between the effects of nitroprusside and nitroglycerin on ischemic injury during acute MI. Circulation *54*:766, 1976.

Khaja F, Walton JA Jr, Brymer JF, Goldstein S, et al: Intracoronary fibrinolytic therapy in acute myocardial infarction: Report of a prospective randomized trial. N Engl J Med *308*:1305, 1983.

Mantle JA, Roberts WJ, Russell RO, Rackley ED: Emergency revascularization for acute myocardial infarction: An unproved experimental approach. Am J Cardiol *44*:1407, 1974.

Myer J, Merx W, Schmitz H, et al: Percutaneous transluminal coronary angioplasty immediately after intracoronary streptolysis of transmural myocardial infarction. Circulation *66*:905, 1982.

Passamani ER: Nitroprusside in myocardial infarction (Editorial). N Engl J Med *306*:1168, 1982.

Rude RE, Muller JE, Braunwald E: Efforts to limit the size of myocardial infarcts. Ann Intern Med *95*:736, 1981.

25

ANTICOAGULANTS, ANTIPLATELET AGENTS, AND BETA-BLOCKERS IN ACUTE ISCHEMIC HEART DISEASE

Anticoagulants in Acute Myocardial Infarction (MI)

Background

Clinical reports in the literature show conflicting effects on acute mortality. This is thought to be largely caused by experimental design or interpretation of results (see Gifford and Feinstein). Routine anticoagulation of the patient with acute MI has enjoyed varying periods of popularity paralleling these reports.

Studies of venous thrombosis in the lower extremities using ^{125}I-labeled fibrinogen show an increased occurrence in patients with acute MI, particularly in the presence of left ventricular failure or cardiogenic shock.

The British Working Party Study and the VA Cooperative Study, as well as a number of smaller investigations, as described in Gifford and Feinstein, have demonstrated that deep vein thrombosis and pulmonary and systemic thromboembolism in patients with acute MI can be reduced with full anticoagulation.

Neither the VA nor the British Working Party studies have shown that anticoagulation prevented or inhibited infarct extension or recurrence. However, several recent papers employing historical control populations have once again suggested that an acute reduction in the mortality rate exists.

Low-dose heparin, used prophylactically, has been shown to be as effective as full anticoagulation in the prevention of venous thrombosis. However, there has not been a large and well-controlled study of MI patients to examine the effects of low-dose heparin on the incidence of mural thrombi or systemic or pulmonary emboli.

Indications

Full-dose anticoagulation for prophylaxis:

(1) For extensive lower extremity varicosities

(2) For left ventricular aneurysm (especially when thrombus can be visualized using noninvasive imaging techniques)

(3) Markedly depressed global left ventricular function with ejection fractions $\leq 25\%$

Low-dose ("mini-dose") therapy for prophylaxis:

For all other patients with acute MI, (in the absence of specific contraindications) particularly those predisposed to venous thrombotic disease of the legs and pelvis; patients with massive obesity, with massive cardiac enlargement, or with severe congestive heart failure.

Method

Heparin is the drug of choice in the acute setting because of its rapid onset of action, ease of control, and rapidity of reversal should bleeding or other complications from therapy arise.

Full anticoagulation:

(1) Loading dose: 5000–10,000 units given by rapid IV infusion

(2) Maintenance dose: 25,000–30,000 units/24 hr, with dose adjusted to keep activated partial thromboplastin time at 2–3 times normal

(3) For LV aneurysm with documented thrombus, anticoagulation should be continued with warfarin until there is evidence by platelet labeling or echocardiography of thrombus dissolution. (Extended anticoagulation in LV aneurysm without demonstrated thrombus or systemic embolization is less compelling but may be indicated when the aneurysm is extensive or cardiac output is low.) Dose: 5–10 mg po initially, then dose sufficient to maintain prothrombin time twice control

Low-dose heparin. Rationale:

(1) Small doses of heparin can prevent thrombin formation, while large doses are required once intravascular coagulation has been initiated.

(2) Because of the lower dose used, the incidence of adverse bleeding is greatly reduced compared with conventional full-dose therapy.

Dose: 5000 units in 0.2 ml of solution every 8–12 hr, given by fine needle (No. 25 or No. 26 gauge) into the subcutaneous fat pad of the abdominal wall. The area should not be rubbed after injection.

The injection site should be rotated. Small areas of ecchymosis at the site of injection can be expected.

Because small doses of heparin are used, follow-up studies of coagulation parameters are not required.

Use of Antiplatelet Agents Following Myocardial Infarction

Mechanisms of Action. Both thrombosis and coronary spasm are thought to participate individually or together in initiating and perpetuating the acute myocardial infarction process; mechanisms, however, remain incompletely understood.

Pathways in Platelet Function (Fig. 25–1). There are two major pathways. One occurs in platelets and results in the production of thromboxane, the other occurs in the vascular endothelium and results in the production of prostacyclin. The pathways counterbalance each other, the former promoting platelet aggregation and

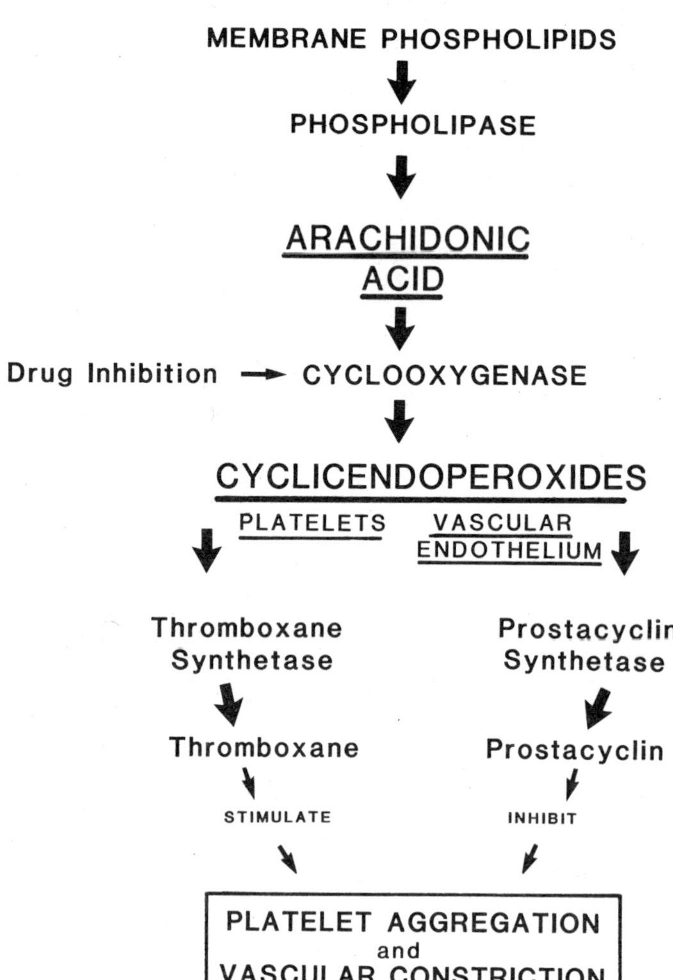

Figure 25–1. Pathways in platelet function.

vascular spasm, the latter inhibiting platelet aggregation and inducing vascular dilation.

In addition, thrombin (resulting from tissue thromboplastin and activation of clotting factor XII) promotes platelet aggregation and (independently) thromboxane A_2 formation.

Pathway Inhibition

Cyclooxygenase Inhibitors

These include aspirin, indomethacin, sulfinpyrazone, phenylbutazone, ibuprofen, and other nonsteroidal antiinflammatory agents.

Aspirin results in reversible cyclooxygenase acetylation in the endothelial cell; acetylation in the platelet, however, is not reversible and occurs at lower doses of aspirin. Lower aspirin doses (half a tablet a day) can therefore block thromboxane without significantly blocking prostacyclin.

Other pathway inhibitors include adrenocorticosteroids (inhibition of phospholipase is the presumed mechanism) and inhibitors of thromboxane synthetase (none in this category have been tested for prevention of thrombosis).

Agents that increase levels of cyclic adenosine monophosphatase (C-AMP) inhibit many platelet functions. Dipyridamole does so by inhibition of platelet phosphodiesterase, impeding the degradation of C-AMP to monophosphatases.

Clinical Usefulness

No benefit has been demonstrated by acute use of platelet-active agents.

For chronic use after acute myocardial infarction:

(1) Aspirin. No decrease in mortality or recurrent myocardial infarction has been found (Aspirin Myocardial Infarction Study—AMIS). Benefit was suggested but not proved with use in the first 6 months after infarction in the Persantine-Aspirin Re-Infarction Study (PARIS).

(2) Sulfinpyrazone. A reduction in sudden death has been reported, but results have been challenged. There appears to be no reduction in mortality rate or recurrent infarction (Anturane Reinfarction Trial).

(3) Dipyridamole. Nonstatistical reduction in mortality rate alone and in combination with aspirin (PARIS), with most reduction in those treated within the first 6 months after infarction.

(4) Other agents. No conclusive clinical trials have been done.

Beta-Blockers

Rationale. Reduce sympathetically induced arrhythmias or ischemia; mechanisms for benefit are only conjectural. They have an additional antiplatelet effect.

Chronic Use after Myocardial Infarction. Large clinical studies have shown reduction of mortality rate (range, 26–40%), sudden death (40% with timolol), and recurrent infarction (23% with timolol) over the 3 year postinfarction period. The major benefit appears to be in the first 1–2 years.

Acute Use after Myocardial Infarction. As noted in Chapter 24, beta-blockers reduce infarct size in experimental animals. However, clinical studies have not conclusively demonstrated significant benefit, and adverse effects may be serious, e.g., cardiac failure.

Dose

Propranolol (Beta-Blocker Heart Attack Trial — BHAT), 60–80 mg tid

Timolol (Norwegian Multicenter Study), 10 mg bid
Metoprolol (Hjalmarson et al), 100 mg bid

Other beta-blockers that require less frequent administration may have similar benefit but have not been prospectively studied. Their chronic use should await the general acceptance of this class of drugs for secondary prevention postinfarction.

Use. In postinfarction patients without contraindication to beta-blockade. They may be given with caution in the presence of mild, compensated heart failure.

All patients derive benefit, although those at greatest risk (previous infarction), and those at moderate risk (hemodynamic complications or markedly elevated cardiac enzymes during index infarction) derive the greatest benefit.

Administration is best begun within 1–4 weeks of the acute infarction and continued for 1–2 years. Benefits of longer treatment have not been evaluated.

REFERENCES

Beta Blocker Heart Attack Trial Research Group: A randomized trial of propranolol in patients with acute MI. JAMA *247*:1707, 1982.

Chalmers TC, Motta RJ, Smith H, Kuntzler AM: Evidence favoring the use of anticoagulants in the hospital phase of acute myocardial infarction. N Engl J Med *297*:1091, 1977.

Gifford RH, Feinstein AR: A critique of methodology of studies of anticoagulant therapy for myocardial infarction. N Engl J Med *280*:351, 1969.

Hjalmarson A, Elmfeldt D, Herlitz J, et al: Effect on mortality of metoprolol in acute myocardial infarction. Lancet *2*:823, 1981.

Norwegian Multicenter Study Group: Timolol-induced reduction in mortality and reinfarction in patients surviving acute MI. N Engl J Med *304*:801, 1981.

Shand DG: Beta adrenergic blocking drugs post acute MI. Mod Conc Cardiovasc Dis *51*:103, 1982.

Winter S, Capone RJ: Drug prevention of myocardial infarction. Res Staff Physician *27*:42, 1981.

V

AFTER THE CCU

26
CARDIAC REHABILITATION

Physiologic and Psychosocial Consequences of Myocardial Infarction

In the aftermath of myocardial infarction, several important questions and issues must be faced by the patient and the family, such as medications, prognosis, job resumption, and sexual intercourse. Following transfer from the Coronary Care Unit to an intermediate care facility or general medical ward, the patient is usually able to begin to come to grips with his or her diagnosis of myocardial infarction. This is an appropriate time to commence the process of cardiac rehabilitation, the object of which is to educate and inform the patient's spouse and family about the cause of infarction and to restore the individual's sense of physical and psychologic well being.

In our experience, a major catalyst in this effort is the *nurse.* Nurses, particularly those with strong educational backgrounds in cardiovascular disease and teaching, are particularly important resources for the patient and family during the critical weeks postinfarction. During this time, appropriate reading material and cassette tapes and movies are extremely beneficial for informing the patient about the illness and its implications. Because nurses have intensive day-to-day contact with patients and are available to interact with patients and families more often than physicians, they are indispensable to the process of in-hospital cardiac rehabilitation.

Many important *activities* of the cardiac patient following myocardial infarction must be considered. Most relate to activity levels, which have been increasingly liberalized in recent years. Although there are no definitive prospective studies, most patients with uncomplicated myocardial infarction (the absence of postinfarct angina, congestive heart failure, important cardiac arrhythmias, or conduction disturbances) appear to do well clinically during early mobilization in the hospital.

There has been an increasing tendency to *discharge* patients with uncomplicated infarctions, including nontransmural infarction, within 10 to 14 days of admission. However, recent evidence suggests that the incidence of significant reinfarction (infarct extension) may complicate as many as 40% of patients who are admitted with an initial nontransmural infarction, and it appears that the issue of early discharge following even an uncomplicated "myocardial infarction" is not yet settled (see also Chapter 7).

Clearly, patients who have had myocardial infarctions complicated by left ventricular failure, shock, arrhythmias, or other medical illnesses should be managed more conservatively and may require a hospitalization of up to 3–4 weeks.

On balance, it appears that *early ambulation* for the uncomplicated myocardial patient is safe. In fact, the debilitating effects of bedrest provide very strong support for its use. Increasing ambulation also provides the physician with an opportunity to observe the patient's effort capacity and symptomatic status postinfarction.

Cardiac Risk Factors

(See also Chapter 3)

Identifying and correcting *risk factors* known to predispose to coronary artery disease are of paramount importance. Patient education about the risks of cigarette smoking, hypertension, elevated serum cholesterol, and dietary habits should be stressed during the recovery phase of infarction. Unfortunately, determinations of cholesterol and triglyceride levels may be spuriously depressed following acute myocardial infarction; unless values are obtained within the first 24 hours after admission (see Chapter 7), an accurate assessment of lipids and lipoproteins cannot be obtained for 6 to 8 weeks postinfarction.

The post-MI recovery period affords a unique opportunity to counsel patients and family members about the adverse effects of cigarette smoking, hypertension, and diabetes mellitus. The recognition and aggressive management of these risk factors may decrease the likelihood for future coronary events, although there is still no consensus that "risk factor modification" alters the natural history of coronary artery disease progression postinfarction.

Activity in the Hospital Postinfarction; Submaximal Exercise Tests

Patients with uncomplicated myocardial infarctions undergo gradually increasing ambulation during their 2 week hospitalization after infarction. In general, short walks around the quarters are encouraged two to three times per day, with increasing duration during the 4 to 5 day time period prior to discharge. In addition, patients are permitted bathroom privileges, including washing and shaving, approximately 4 to 5 days postinfarction. Taking a tepid or warm shower during the second week postinfarction is permitted in patients with uncomplicated infarction. Patients with complicated myocardial infarctions or those who develop postinfarct angina may be kept at more restricted activity levels until their complications abate.

Prior to discharge (2 to 4 weeks postinfarction), we recommend a *submaximal treadmill test* (maximum heart rate, approximately 120 beats per minute) in patients with uncomplicated infarction.

Several retrospective and prospective studies have indicated that exercise testing early after myocardial infarction is both safe and efficacious. The major impact of submaximal stress testing is its prognostic value for predicting subsequent coronary events and sudden death. Both short-term and long-term follow-up studies indicate a higher incidence of subsequent myocardial infarction and mortality in patients who exhibit ST segment depression, compared with groups of individuals who do not display ST segment depression. In addition, angina that develops during submaximal exercise testing also has been shown to have predictive value for patients who are likely to develop angina during the ensuing year.

Moreover, an exercise test prior to discharge is important for formulating patient guidelines for exercise at home, reassuring him of his physical status, and determining his risk of complications. Finally, the psychologic impact of good performance on the exercise test may have a favorable effect on recovery and well being.

We routinely recommend that a patient with an uncomplicated myocardial infarction undergo a submaximal treadmill test prior to discharge, *and if this test is performed without angina, ST segment change, or significant ventricular arrhythmia,* the patient is permitted to commence walking one fourth to one half mile per day. If a patient develops angina, ST segment changes, or arrhythmias, medical therapy (beta-blockers with or without long-acting nitrates) is initiated. As a corollary, patients who display an abnormal treadmill response during submaximal predischarge stress testing should not increase their activity level until there is confirmation of improvement upon a subsequent exercise test 1 to 2 months later.

If a patient has a *strongly* positive submaximal treadmill test following MI (defined as ≥ 1.5–2.0 mm ST depression in ECG leads remote from the infarct area, or severe chest pain), we recommend *urgent cardiac catheterization* to define coronary anatomy, preferably prior to discharge. An alternative approach is to maximize medical therapy (beta-blockers/nitrates/calcium channel blockers), limit physical activity postdischarge, and subsequently readmit the patient within 2–4 weeks for elective cardiac catheterization.

At 4 to 6 weeks following discharge, the patient with an uncomplicated infarction (or without provokable ischemia by submaximal stress testing) is permitted to resume *sexual activity.* Six weeks after discharge, the patient is permitted to walk one half to 1 mile per day and may begin driving an auto on a limited basis.

Six to eight weeks following discharge, the patient with an uncomplicated infarction may *return to work,* preferably on a half-time basis for 1 to 2 weeks until it is clear that he or she has not experienced recurrent symptoms or undue fatigue.

Posthospital Cardiac Rehabilitation

Provided the postinfarction patient has not developed postinfarct angina or objective evidence for provokable myocardial ischemia by stress testing, a program of regular *supervised physical activity* is encouraged. Although not all patients are suitable for this type of activity (nor do all patients desire to engage in a physical training program), the potential benefits of cardiac rehabilitation by a medically supervised exercise program are noteworthy. The benefits of cardiac rehabilitation include improved hemodynamic, physiologic, symptomatic, and psychologic status. The results of several retrospective and prospective studies that have examined the physiologic benefits of supervised exercise indicate that cardiac patients have improved exercise tolerance and can perform more physical labor before fatigue or symptoms occur, after an exercise training program. Furthermore, the heart rate and blood pressure response to any fixed work load, and consequently the myocardial oxygen demand, are reduced after exercise training so that there is less chance of the patient developing cardiac ischemia. The treatment of myocardial infarction, including bedrest, results in a marked decrease of physical work tolerance. Exercise training reverses this decrease. The end result is that exercise-trained patients can perform more household and occupational tasks more comfortably. This permits a more rapid return to a normal lifestyle, with accompanying psychologic benefits.

The psychologic benefits of exercise training have not been as comprehensively studied as have the physiologic benefits. Nevertheless, there is general agreement that patients participating in such activity have reduced anxiety and depression, as well as increased self-esteem and a more positive perception of personal health status. It is unclear whether the psychologic benefit results from the exercise per se, or from the group interaction.

Individual prospective controlled studies have failed to demonstrate any decrease in morbidity and mortality in patients adhering to an exercise program. However, May et al have recently reviewed all randomized controlled trials of exercise therapy after myocardial infarction. Only studies using a randomized design and enrolling more than 100 patients were examined. Although nonc of the exercise trials showed a statistically significant reduction in total mortality, all but one had a positive trend favoring the physical training group, which varied from 21 to 32%. The trials were all too small to test the hypothesis that exercise reduces overall mortality, as they were not designed with this as the primary endpoint.

Of the six exercise studies, involving 2752 patients, five showed a reduction in mortality. Pooling of the results indicated that the six studies are consistent with a 19% reduction in total mortality in the intervention group, which is statistically significant ($P < .05$). This result suggests that exercise training is nearly as effective as prophylactic beta-blockade on postmyocardial infarction mortality.

Although this result is encouraging, there are inherent statistical problems with the pooling of different studies, and as yet there is no *definite* proof that exercise therapy improves the morbidity or mortality statistics for any post-MI patient group.

Despite the lack of consensus regarding reinfarction and mortality, it appears that a medically supervised cardiac rehabilitation program places the patient at no increased risk, and the broad-based qualitative improvement experienced by many patients strongly supports its use.

REFERENCES

Davidson DM, DeBusk RF: Prognostic value of a single exerise test 3 weeks after uncomplicated myocardial infarction. Circulation *61*:236, 1980.

Hutter AM, Sidel VW, Shine KI, et al: Early hospital discharge after myocardial infarction. N Engl J Med *288*:1141, 1973.

Marmor A, Sobel BE, Roberts R: Factors presaging early recurrent myocardial infarction ("extension"). Am J Cardiol *48*:603, 1981.

May GS, Furberg CD, Eberlein KA, et al: Secondary prevention after myocardial infarction: A review of short-term acute phase trials. Prog Cardiovasc Dis *25*:335, 1983.

Pollock ML, Schmidt DH: Heart Disease and Rehabilitation. Boston, Houghton Mifflin, 1979.

Theroux P, Waters DD, Halphen C, et al: Prognostic value of exercise testing soon after myocardial infarction. N Engl J Med *301*:341, 1979.

Turner JD, Rogers WJ, Mantle JA, et al: Coronary angiography soon after myocardial infarction. Chest *77*:58, 1980.

Wenger NK: Exercise and the Heart. Philadelphia, F.A. Davis, 1978.

Wenger NK, Hellerstein HK: Rehabilitation of the Coronary Patient. New York, John Wiley & Sons, 1978.

Page numbers in italics indicate illustrations;
t following page numbers indicates a table.